THE FIRST CLINICALLY PROVEN
EATING PLAN TO END
OUR NATION'S SECRET EPIDEMIC

Inflammation
Nation

Floyd H. "Ski" Chilton, Ph.D.

with Laura Tucker

A Fireside Book
Published by Simon & Schuster

New York   London   Toronto   Sydney

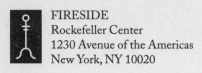

FIRESIDE
Rockefeller Center
1230 Avenue of the Americas
New York, NY 10020

For information regarding special discounts for bulk purchases,
please contact Simon & Schuster Special Sales:
1-800-456-6798 or business@simonandschuster.com

Designed by Ruth Lee Mui

Manufactured in the United States of America

10 9 8 7 6 5 4 3 2 1

Library of Congress Cataloging-in-Publication Data
Chilton, Floyd H.
    Inflammation nation : the first clinically proven eating plan to end our
nation's secret epidemic / by Floyd H. Chilton with Laura Tucker.
      p.   cm.
Includes bibliographical references and index.
    1. Inflammation—Popular works.   2. Inflammation—Diet therapy.
I. Tucker, Laura.   II. Title.
RB131.C486   2005
616'.0473—dc22   2004056402

ISBN 0-7432-6964-0

This book is dedicated to my son, Josh,
and my father, Floyd,
for their inspiring examples of
extraordinary courage.

Contents

Part 3: Tools for Healthy Living

Acknowledgments

First and foremost, I would like to acknowledge my God for his continuous love and guidance. I would like to honor my children, Candice, Josh, Shane, and Sarah, for continually providing purpose to my life. I would like to express deep appreciation to my mom, for her unwavering strength and support, and to my sisters, Tammy and Tanya, for being my biggest fans! I thank Karen Guedella for her title inspiration, and thank her and Mark Palmer for first believing in the foundations of this book. Dr. Cash McCall reminded me constantly that if I was true to myself, everything else would fall into place, and Briana Laurene believed unflaggingly that this book would change people's lives. I am grateful for the inspiration of both of these dear friends.

I will forever be grateful to my friend and agent, Laurie Bernstein, for believing in and guiding me from the very beginning of this project, and for introducing me to my one-of-a-kind cowriter, Laura Tucker, who partnered with me for the most creative adventure I have ever experienced. It has been a wonderful collaboration. Thanks to Linda Easter, M.S., R.D., L.D.N., who with ProNutra (Viocare Technologies, Inc.) helped me to implement the Chilton Program; to Eric Sherertz for his inspirational illustrations; and to Carol Colman and Carol Mann.

Gratitude to numerous friends and colleagues, including Tim Childress, Dr. Bob Sherertz, Dr. Brad Undem, Debra Marshall, Scott Derks, Dr. Jon Arm, Jim Morgan, Bill Lee, Gary Lackey, Cindy Sally, Dr. Jim Smith, Dr. Bill Applegate, Margaret Urquhart, Rev. Sheldon McCarter, Rev. Jerry Webb, Rev. John Hamilton, Teika York, Frank Sajovic, and Dr. Kristin Anstrom for their unconditional care and support; and to Ted, Cindy, and all my friends in Charleston for providing strength at a very critical time. Many thanks to Dr. Kevin High and Dr. Mark Payne for helping me with the Inflammatory Quotient Quiz.

I was incredibly blessed to have been trained by four of the best fatty-acid scientists in the world: Dr. Roger Lumb, at Western Carolina University; Dr. Robert Wykle, at Wake Forest University School of Medicine; Dr. Robert Murphy, at National Jewish Center Medical and Research Center; and Dr. Lawrence Lichtenstein, at Johns Hopkins University School of Medicine. Thank you for allowing me to stand on your shoulders.

I would like to acknowledge the National Institutes of Health for twenty years of funding research in my laboratory, and the laboratories of others whose science inspired this book.

Laura and I would both like to express deep appreciation for the professionalism of the whole Simon & Schuster team: Trish Todd, Mark Gompertz, Marcia Burke, Loretta Denner, and Nora Reichard, and especially our editor, Cherise Davis, for her serenity, faith, and good counsel along the way.

Laura would also like to thank her family, the Tuckers and the Crowells, for all their help and patience—especially Doug and Lily.

The principles that guide this book were derived from the results of thousands of basic and clinical scientific studies, and it could not have been written without the contribution of those scientists, and the anonymous contribution of their students, postdoctoral fellows, collaborators, and reviewers. Thanks go to them, and to everyone who continues to work to advance these ideas.

Foreword
Charles E. McCall, M.D.

Over forty years ago, a young man with shock, fever, and pneumonia was brought by ambulance to Cambridge City Hospital, Massachusetts, where I became his attending physician—for a short time. Within twelve hours after his admission, the patient, still in the prime of his life, was dead. My brief attempts to help him had been futile; the outcome of his illness was likely predetermined long before he'd entered the hospital.

This tragic event, which happened during my training as a physician and specialist in infectious diseases and inflammation at Harvard Medical School, shook me deeply. I felt helpless, and rushed to the medical school library in an attempt to understand the reason for my patient's untimely death. I noted that his white blood cells, when viewed under a microscope, were stippled with bizarre, angry-looking, abnormal granules. I soon found that these cells are called "toxic" leukocytes, an abnormality defined at the turn of the twentieth century. In my patient, the word *toxic*, which means poisoned, was fitting.

A widespread inflammatory process, attempting to eradicate an infection, had turned instead upon its keeper. Rather than curing my patient, the inflammatory process killed him, by disrupting the function of his vital organs. In essence, his body had committed suicide. This seems astonishing, but it is true. This frightening, humbling, and baffling encounter with the double-edged sword of inflammation—both helper and villain—charted the course of my career as a physician scientist in the field of inflammatory diseases.

Some four decades later, I still study inflammation, which I now think of as a gift from Nature that is not always welcome. Such is the nature of the beast. Inflammation is as old as human and animal history, existing in fossil evidence. It is described in the first written communications of humans. Indeed, as I remind the medical students I lecture, the first description of a specific disease process is inflammation. The Sumerian pictorial writings of seven thousand years ago display a "bier," or flame, to describe the scorching associated with wounds to the body. Early Egyptian, Chinese, and Greek writing also included descriptions of and symbols for the features of inflammation, such as heat, redness, swelling, and pain.

We have each one of us experienced inflammation by the time we can walk and talk: tenderness, swelling, redness, and local heat around a cut, for instance. When inflammation is chronic, other generalized features come to the forefront: chronic fatigue, vague muscle pains, poor appetite, occasional weight loss, sleepiness, and even depression. These systemic effects of inflammation are frequent visitors to those with primary inflammatory diseases such as rheumatoid arthritis, lupus, inflammatory diseases of the bowel, and hepatitis.

My patients with inflammatory diseases can be sick unto rapid death, chronically maimed and disabled—or completely unaware of the destructive process that simmers among their various organs and tissues as they wrestle with a friend turned enemy.

To make the bad news worse, inflammatory processes like atherosclerosis, Alzheimer's, and dementia may remain completely hidden for many years. They hold their secrets, and when they confess, the game may be just about over. Clinical medicine continues its quest for surrogate markers to sniff out those secrets and to track the epidemic of inflammation, but the results are slow in coming. In this book, Dr. Chilton rightly admonishes us to take rational steps now to stem the tide.

Inflammation Nation captures the unique challenge that inflammation poses to our health, and provides an approach for muting its effects. First, Dr. Chilton convincingly identifies the epidemic of inflammation, whose attack rate for many diseases (asthma, atherosclerosis, arthritis, psoriasis, diabetes, and inflammatory bowel disease, to mention just a few) continues to rise, despite medical progress in understanding and treating many forms of inflammation.

Although less evident to the public than our conspicuous epidemic of obesity, this epidemic of diseases of inflammation is no less serious. From his experiences as a world-class scientist, Dr. Chilton clearly explains the way cells and tissue fluids communicate the messages of inflammation using chemicals as their method.

Dr. Chilton then identifies a causal force behind the epidemic rise in these diseases, by providing evidence for a major contributor to the epidemic: the constituents of the food in the Western world's diet. *We are what we eat,* and this terrible foe sneaks in through our gut to modify the very nature of our inflammatory engine, the same way our gasoline carburetors, running "too rich," will eventually result in a dysfunctional engine.

Finally, *Inflammation Nation* gives hope to sufferers by providing a well-conceived approach to limit the devastation of the destructive effects of out-of-control inflammation on our health. This all-natural dietary approach works like medication, but with none of the side effects or expense of the drugs we ordinarily rely upon to treat our patients. And this approach does not carry a risk of compromising the beneficial side of inflammation, like most of the drugs we physicians use to treat inflammatory diseases.

Throughout all sections of the book, Dr. Chilton emphasizes outcomes and preventive medicine in the field of nutrition, reminding us of the ultimate quest of medical practice: not only to diagnose and treat, but to predict negative outcomes, and to avoid them whenever possible.

Forty years later, I remain fascinated and puzzled by the whole business of inflammation and its companion diseases. We have entered the era of genomics now—how exciting this is, for scientists like me! Good genes, bad genes, and indifferent genes all have input into the diseases of inflammation. But there is a risk in putting all of our eggs into this basket. Our environment is at least of equal importance, and, as Dr. Chilton emphasizes, the epidemic of inflammation has outraced genetic changes, leaving the environment as the major determinant in this epidemic, specifically our readily available, delicious, and affordable food. Our food industries cleverly serve our habits. What are we to do, and when?

A television commercial reminds us that it is not the idea that counts at the end of the day, but the action taken on that idea. Research medicine is rightly criticized for forgetting who is coming for dinner, for not trans-lating discoveries and new information into action that relieves the human plight. Dr. Chilton, in *Inflammation Nation,* has not stopped with descriptive information, but takes a bold step into advocacy. He provides information, upon which he constructs an action plan. He is persuasive, and his message both makes sense and is practical. It is worthy of our attention, for what we eat helps make us what we are.

PART 1

The
Secret Epidemic

Introduction

A **silent plague is sweeping America,** and the vast majority of us are at risk. It has taken the form of a statistically significant and incalculably devastating series of epidemics—an "epidemic of epidemics."

I believe this plague is largely preventable, and yet we are doing little to stop its spread. On the contrary, we're actually encouraging a tidal wave of disease. At best, these illnesses compromise our quality of life; at worst, they can be painful, debilitating, and fatal.

Consider the following:

◆ Seventy million Americans suffer from arthritis—or *one in every three adults.* That's *twice* as many arthritis sufferers as there were two decades ago.*

◆ More than 20 million Americans have asthma today. It is the *sixth* most common chronic human disease.

◆ More than 50 million Americans suffer every year from allergies, a number that has doubled in the past twenty years. There has been a 100 percent increase in the prevalence of hay fever in developed countries in each of the last three decades. Allergic dermatitis affects us at *triple* the rate in 1960. Ten percent of our young children are affected by allergic dermatitis.

◆ There were 18.2 million people in the United States with diabetes in 2002, a 49 percent increase from ten years ago. This debilitating disease contributes to about two hundred thousand deaths in the United States each year.

◆ Cardiovascular disease is the number one killer of Americans. Almost *64 million* Americans have it in some form, and it killed almost a million people in 2001.

* Source: Arthritis Foundation

Inflammatory Diseases in the United States

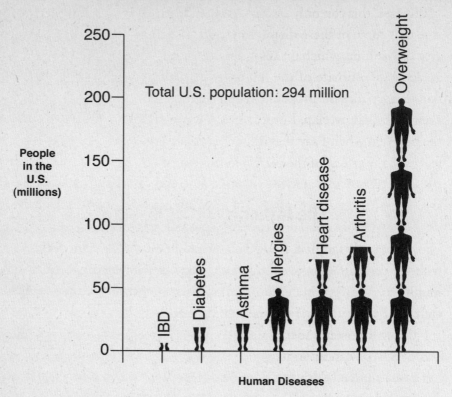

- ◆ Eczema is the most common skin condition in children under eleven; an estimated 15 million people in the United States suffer from the symptoms of this disease.
- ◆ One million Americans have inflammatory bowel disease.

Anyone would agree that these numbers are overwhelming. But they're even more devastating when you realize that this isn't just a random laundry list of conditions. In fact, these diseases all share a single underlying cause.

What's the common denominator linking these seemingly disparate diseases, and other serious ones, including lupus, Crohn's disease, and psoriasis? The answer comes from a surprising quarter: the body's own self-defense system. These are all *inflammatory diseases*, diseases that occur when the body's own defense system turns against itself.

And our bodies are turning against themselves in record numbers. Each one of these diseases, taken individually, represents a serious health problem in this country. Taken together, as a category of diseases, this can only be seen as a pandemic. It is true that some of these diseases overlap, like allergies and asthma, which makes it difficult to make an accurate estimate of the full scope of the inflammatory disease problem in this country. But even with that overlap, I don't think I'm overstating the problem when I say that inflammatory diseases affect as many as *half* of the people in this country.

> Almost 50 percent of Americans suffer from an inflammatory disease.

The Inflammatory Cluster

You're probably familiar, from the news and movies like *Erin Brockovich*, with the phenomenon called the "cancer cluster," when people in a community or a profession develop related types of cancer in disproportionately high percentages. It's an absolutely terrifying occurrence.

When a cluster is identified, researchers immediately look for a proximate cause, a cancer-inducing agent to which every one of the patients has been exposed. When that proximate cause is uncovered (a factory dumping toxic chemicals into the groundwater, for example), the rest of us thank our lucky stars that it didn't happen in *our* neighborhood.

When I began my research into the connection between diet and inflammatory disease, I was simply searching for something to help people who suffered from advanced and chronic inflammatory disease. I wanted to find a natural, dietary solution that would alleviate symptoms in people who had otherwise exhausted their options. But I came to realize, as I hope you will over the course of this book, that the problem of inflammatory disease was much, much bigger than I had thought—and the stakes much higher as a result.

In fact, the soaring rise in inflammatory disease in this country is nothing less than a cluster in its own right. It's a nationwide cluster, a cluster without walls, unbounded by the typical limits of geography or demographics. You *can't* breathe a sigh of relief that you live outside the radius of the toxic-waste spill, because there is no "outside." There is no localized danger zone, no limited area that can be cordoned off and sanitized.

It is when we begin to look for the proximate cause of this tremendous, nationwide epidemic that the terrible gravity of the situation hits home: the answer may in fact be right on our dinner plates. I believe that a major component driving these diseases is our diet, and the "toxic-waste spill," to continue the metaphor, is *our very food supply*. There is no safe house, no place to hide, unless we fundamentally change the way we eat, in the ways prescribed in this book.

> A major component driving these diseases is our food supply.

This disaster has sneaked up on us, but not overnight: the circumstances leading up to it have been brewing for a century or more. The staggering number of Americans suffering from these painful and debilitating diseases are, horribly, acting as the canaries in the coal mine. Their agony is sending a message, loud and clear, to those of us who have so far managed to dodge the bullet. This book isn't about the division between people who have inflammatory disease and people who don't. It's not about "who has it" and "who doesn't"; instead it's about "who doesn't" and "who *will?*" Every single one of us has pulled a chair up to this contaminated trough—which means that *every single one of us* is at risk.

"Why Haven't I Heard About This?"

You're probably wondering: if out-of-control inflammation is a silent plague threatening all of us, and not just a rare and exotic condition that affects the unfortunate few, why don't I know about it?

In fact, you know more about inflammation than you think. Like oxygen, inflammation is essential to our continued survival. When the inflammation system goes off course, we quickly turn to medication; I'd bet that there isn't a soul among us who doesn't have a bottle of aspirin in the medicine cabinet. This wonder drug quiets pain, soothes fever, and reduces swelling, like several of the other very effective anti-inflammatory drugs on the market.

Sometimes, however, our system becomes chronically inflamed. *Why* this happens is a puzzle. But we've been gathering the pieces of this puzzle for a while. Pharmaceutical companies have played an important role in uncovering the mysteries of how the inflammation system works. In fact, I like to refer to the inflammatory pathway that is the subject of this book as "the billion-dollar pathway," because it has absorbed more time and research—and research dollars—than almost any other area of medicine in the last thirty years. Soon, you will know it by another name: the AA Pathway (more about this later). The ability to block the AA Pathway is the magic behind blockbuster drugs like Celebrex and Singulair, as well as aspirin and other nonsteroidal anti-inflammatory drugs (NSAIDs). The AA Pathway is also the magic behind the Chilton Program, a whole new all-natural way of thinking about inflammation.

Why the Stakes Are So High Right Now

The shockingly high number of people who have been diagnosed with inflammatory disease is one reason that we must come to terms with this plague. The fact that every single one of us is potentially in the line of fire is another. But out-of-control inflammation looms large as a public health issue for a variety of other reasons as well:

◆ Inflammatory diseases are debilitating and, in many cases, fatal. And there is no cure for these diseases. Although in most cases, we've gotten better at treating their symptoms, treatment often means expensive, long-term medications with side effects that can be as damaging as the diseases themselves, and even the best medications don't work all the time, or for everybody.

◆ More diseases have inflammation at their root than we think. Inflammation, it turns out, is the culprit behind many of the life-threatening conditions we thought were closed cases. For instance, ten years ago, cardiologists thought elevated blood lipids like cholesterol and triglycerides were the primary cause of heart disease, so we categorized atherosclerosis as a lipid-storage disease. Now we believe that heart disease, the leading killer of Americans, actually has inflammation at its root. And new research shows that underlying inflammation may be linked to other major killers, like Alzheimer's and certain types of cancer.

◆ Other human conditions have a significant inflammatory component. Even conditions that aren't strictly categorized as inflammatory diseases frequently have a significant inflammatory component, which is often the root of chronic pain and

deforming tissue damage. For example, inflammation is a major driving force behind type 2 diabetes and dementia. In fact, inflammation may play a major role in
the category of ailments and diseases we have previously called "aging." Consequently, treating and preventing inflammation can mean a tremendous boon for all
of us, often resulting in an enormous increase in function and great relief from
pain.

◆ Inflammation isn't the only burgeoning epidemic. Approximately 64 percent of
Americans are overweight or obese. Not only does being overweight exacerbate
an existing inflammatory disease, but fat cells play a major role in the creation of
the messengers that cause inflammatory disease.

◆ More and more people are affected every year. Today's inflammatory disease statistics are alarming. Tomorrow's numbers will be worse. The number of people suffering from these diseases—and dying from them—continues to grow. Our medical
systems, medicines, and technologies have never been better or more accessible to
many people, and yet these diseases flourish as if we lived in the Dark Ages.

If we hope to see any meaningful relief from this pandemic, we must
begin to address its underlying cause; and, to do that, we must investigate
why these diseases are happening to us in such disproportionately high
numbers, and what we're doing that's causing those numbers to rise.

Tammy's Story: A Personal Crusade

Vital journeys in life often start with the intense desire to help someone
whom you love. If almost 50 percent of Americans have an inflammatory
disease, then certainly every American's life has been touched by this epidemic, and I am no exception. It was my own personal experience with
inflammatory diseases in people whom I cared about that motivated me
to dedicate my life to this research.

My sister Tammy was diagnosed with juvenile rheumatoid arthritis
(RA) at the age of thirteen. I truly believe that if Satan were to design a
disease, it would be this one—an opinion that's shared by those who live
with RA, and the doctors who treat it. It's truly a monstrous affliction:
an incurable disease characterized by excruciating pain and gradual debil-
itation.

Tammy is one of the bravest people I've ever met. Although she's been suffering from this demon of a disease since childhood, I don't think I've ever heard her complain—but the physical evidence of her disease is written all over her body. By the age of thirty, her hands were so grotesquely deformed that it hurt just to look at them, and her knees were enormously swollen with bony protuberances, places where the chronic inflammation had affected so much tissue that the shape of the joint was permanently damaged.

To control her disease, Tammy had progressively moved up to more and more serious medications. By the fall of 1997, she was taking a medication called methotrexate, originally designed as an anti-cancer drug. It is very powerful and toxic. The immediate side effects included mouth sores, diarrhea, and a loss of appetite, but there was also a long-term threat: taken in high enough concentrations for long periods of time, methotrexate can eventually threaten every major organ system in the body.

The medication was expensive, the side effects made her very uncomfortable, and, as the mother of three small children, she was worried about its effects on her future health. But like many RA patients, Tammy simply didn't have a choice. This drug was her only hope. The worst part was that the methotrexate wasn't even all that effective. Despite this heavy-duty medication, Tammy still couldn't walk up a flight of stairs or tie her own shoes. And no matter what she did, her disease continued to worsen.

After two full knee replacements and five surgeries to rehabilitate and replace the joints in her hands, Tammy was at the end of her rope. She had heard in RA sufferer support groups an excited buzz about "alternative therapies" promising increased function and pain reduction. The possibility of help was tantalizing, but inaccessible—there was absolutely no consensus about what worked! Some sufferers were claiming terrific results from diets that contained supposedly anti-inflammatory foods, and from taking huge doses of antioxidant vitamins and fatty-acid supplements. Dosages varied wildly, depending on whom you asked, and nobody seemed to be all that concerned about science or safety.

Understandably overwhelmed by the contradictory information whizzing back and forth, Tammy called me. At the time, I was a faculty member at the prestigious Johns Hopkins Asthma and Allergy Center and an internationally recognized expert in asthma.

"I need to try something else," she said. "My doctor is telling me I've exhausted my options, but what I'm doing clearly isn't working, and I can't go on like this. Isn't there anything else I can do?"

"I have no idea," I said. "But don't you *dare* take anything until I do."

That night, I spent the evening at our medical library examining the claims behind these alternative medicines. Tammy had been right: there was a whole culture of people with inflammatory diseases of all kinds, clamoring for help. In almost all cases, their diseases were chronic and progressive. The prescription medications they were taking often had unacceptable side effects, and they were legitimately afraid of the effects these medications might have on their long-term health. Traditional medicine was not providing acceptable solutions for these people, and they were desperate for answers from other quarters.

But if there was help to be found, it wasn't going to be from natural-product companies, which seemed to prey on the hopes and fears of despairing sufferers, trading in great promises that could only end up in profound disappointment. I was appalled by the misinformation about diet and supplements I was reading in the materials I found. At best, the information was useless, the "prescriptions" not much better than snake oil. At worst, the recommendations were downright dangerous—combinations of supplements at dosage levels that could have potentially fatal results, like platelet stickiness and heart attack.

At the same time, I couldn't dismiss everything I found as quackery. As silly as some of the scientific claims were, I could also see the gleam of real treasure there. Sure that I wasn't the only scientist to make these inquiries, I went to Medline, a list of about 11 million references from medical journals, to see what the medical community had to offer. I looked for clinical trials designed to test alternative therapies for inflammatory disease.

Unfortunately, what I found there wasn't much more conclusive. There weren't a lot of studies, and, for the most part, the ones I did find lacked real scientific vigor. Many of them hadn't used a placebo control group, which meant that there wasn't a real standard against which to compare their results. Most of them hadn't taken place in a major medical center setting, where the researchers could ensure strict compliance. And in some cases, there was a question about how the outcomes had been measured. From a scientific perspective, the research was inadequate, to say the least.

But again, there was just enough possibility to intrigue me. There was a large body of evidence indicating a connection between inflammatory disease and diet—specifically, the fatty acids in our diet, which happened to be my own primary area of expertise.

I sat up for several long and sleepless nights thinking about Tammy's options, and my own. At the time, I had two major grants funded by the National Institutes of Health, and I was consulting for three major pharmaceutical companies. In other words, I had a lot of research money at my disposal. I was a world-recognized scientist, specializing in the way that fatty acids are metabolized in the body on a cellular level, and it was very clear from the research I'd found that there was overlap between my field of expertise and inflammation.

As the sun came up on my last sleepless night, I realized I had an opportunity to help my sister, and millions of people like her. Wasn't it time that I started looking at the forest, instead of so closely focusing on the trees?

And so it was that with my colleagues at Johns Hopkins (and building on the work of countless scientists and researchers before me), I began my quest to develop safe, effective, scientifically based, natural approaches to preventing and treating inflammatory disease through diet.

Now I believe I know a major reason why America and other first-world nations are falling prey to the epidemic rise in these diseases despite our unprecedented medical advances. And with that answer in hand, I was able to devise a program—a simple, easy-to-follow diet solution that I believe will help stop, reverse, and even prevent the debilitating effects of an immune system that has been set permanently on overdrive.

Although the program was not designed to supplant medication, it did in some of the patients who were a part of the six clinical trials that tested the foundations of these diet plans. People suffering from inflam-

matory disease often saw a conspicuous difference in the markers of inflammation within *just seven to ten days*.

After following the rules of my dietary program for a month, a
woman with chronic pulmonary disease was able to sleep without oxygen
for the first time in a decade. A lifelong asthmatic and amateur cyclist
achieved a new personal best in cycling, two months after he'd been convinced he'd have to park his bike for good. My oldest son, Josh, who used
to gauge how well he was controlling his asthma by the number of foot-
ball practices and games he missed, hasn't missed one in over a year. And,
after six months on the diet, my own sister opened and closed her hand
completely, for the first time since she was fourteen years old.

How to Use This Book

I have written this book because I believe that we can—safely and naturally—attack this "epidemic of epidemics" where it stands. I believe we
can limit and indeed, in some cases, even reverse the damage it has already done in the lives of so many Americans. I believe that every one of
us is at risk of developing inflammatory disease unless we bring these
fatty acids back into balance. And I know that people who suffer from inflammatory disease can see measurable, and in many cases life-changing,
improvement in their disease, simply by changing what they eat. This,
obviously, makes for a tremendous improvement in their quality of life.

I've designed this book with that end in mind. In the first half of this
book, we'll discuss this silent epidemic. You'll learn how the standard
American diet has led to this crisis of truly enormous proportion.

In the second half of the book, I'll give you the tools you need to fight
back. We'll determine your "Inflammatory Quotient"—your inflammatory risk profile, which will, in turn, determine how you proceed through
the rest of the program. If you have already been diagnosed with an inflammatory disease, or have a strong genetic predisposition in that direc-
tion, you'll follow the Inflammation Solution Diet. This program is *not*
intended to supplant the treatment plan your doctor has put in place, but
to complement it, and I know that both you and your doctor will be
thrilled to note how quickly you see improvement using this plan.

Even if you don't suffer from one of these diseases, you are neverthe-less at significant risk, in part due to your diet. Thus, the other tier of the Chilton Program, the Inflammation Prevention Diet, is designed to ben-efit people who want to do all they can to resist or hold inflammatory dis-ease at bay for themselves and their families.

The Good News

While the Chilton Program represents a radical new way to control in-flammation, it doesn't require a radical adjustment in your ability to enjoy food. The foods you'll find in this program are ordinary and delicious American table foods. I've provided you with four weeks of meal plans for the Solution Program, and four weeks of meal plans for the Prevention Program, so that you can see how easy it is to choose the healthiest and least-inflammatory foods. After that month is over, I believe that you'll look and feel significantly better.

And in this book, you'll find all the tools you'll need to incorporate your new anti-inflammatory eating habits into the rest of your life, long after you've eaten your way through the meal plans. You'll find all the information you need to follow the Chilton Program in easy-to-understand indexes and a new anti-inflammatory nutritional pyramid, so that you can choose delicious, healthy, anti-inflammatory foods at a glance.

The Chilton Program is simple in part because I've designed a new index system that assigns an inflammatory potential value to the most common foods in our food supply. I have called this the Inflammatory Index. These values will enable you, for the first time, to take control of your overactive inflammation by eating foods low on the Inflammation Index. The innovative and easy-to-understand Inflammation Index in this book ensures that anti-inflammatory choices are never farther away than your fingertips.

My research has also indicated that you can't affect inflammation by fatty acids alone: you must also pay close attention to the amount, and types, of carbohydrates you consume. Consequently, reducing the amount of carbohydrates you eat is another cornerstone of the Chilton

Program. It's also one of the reasons that following the prescriptive weight-loss portion of this program can help you lose weight (as other lower-carbohydrate diets like Atkins and South Beach have done), if that's something you need to do. However, there's one enormous difference: the other low-carb diets do not take inflammation into account.

> **Most low-carb diets recommend very pro-inflammatory foods.**

I have nothing but respect for these diets because they have successfully tackled some of America's biggest misconceptions about food. But I am concerned that many of their recommendations may be worsening our epidemic of inflammatory disease.

The Glycemic Index is the gold standard for measuring how different foods affect blood sugar, and it is used extensively by nutritionists. You'll find a ranking that takes that index into account in this book so you can ensure that your carbohydrate intake isn't sabotaging the work you're doing to suppress inflammation on the fatty-acid side.

The Promise

With *Inflammation Nation,* you're really getting two books in one: an explanation of an epidemic, and a very specific dietary takeaway that will help you prevent, treat, and reverse inflammatory disease in your own life and in the lives of those you care about.

Too many Americans suffer from these painful, debilitating diseases. Too many Americans like me have helplessly watched their loved ones fight the uphill battle against them. And every single one of us is at great risk unless we start right now, by changing what we eat and what we feed our families.

Keep reading. You will learn how inflammation, a natural and vital process, works against you; how you can take the first steps to prevent your body's natural defense system from turning against itself; how you can incorporate a more healthful, anti-inflammatory way of eating into your life; and how, in so doing, you can take part in beating back this epidemic of very destructive diseases.

Chapter One
Diagnosis: Affluenza

Carol stands waiting at the doorway. She rubs her sweaty palms against her jeans and checks the hallway clock again. It's 4:02 in the afternoon, and there's still no sign of Tim.

An eternity later, she sees his tiny frame round the corner. She runs down to the end of the driveway to meet him, her terror giving way to relief and anger. "Tim! We checked the pollen count this morning! You know you can't afford to be outside! Where were you?"

Most mothers would kill to have a kid who chose soccer over violent video games and stupid sitcom reruns. But for Carol's severely asthmatic son, running around outside on this gorgeous, early spring day is like swimming in toxic sludge.

Tim coughs for the first time as they're sitting down to dinner. Maybe he's coming down with something, she consoles herself, fooling nobody—she knows that hoarse bark is an asthma cough. By dessert, the whole family can tell it's going to be a long night.

They're not going to go down without a fight. Tim takes his battery of medications, even though the steroids probably won't have enough time to prevent an attack. Carol sets the kitchen timer so he can take another puff of his beta-agonist the second he's permitted to have another dose. Tim sits in the bathroom with the shower running hot for as long as he can take it, and he does his homework in the cloud of the vaporizer. Then it's bedtime, and the cough seems to be getting a little better—or is it? Carol rubs Vicks VapoRub on his chest, more to combat her feeling of helplessness than because she believes it'll do anything.

Asthma is nocturnal, so Carol is, too. She lurks outside Tim's room, her own breath catching with every one of his coughs. At about 3:00 A.M., she hears it—the horrible, hollow, rattling gasp that means her son is desperately struggling for a breath. She doesn't need to pull up his pajama top to see him "pulling," sucking his diaphragm deep into his abdomen in his fight for air.

Her husband is already on the phone with the emergency room, letting them know they're on the way. Praying under her breath, Carol hoists Tim into her arms and runs down the stairs to the waiting car.

I began this book with a list of statistics about the prevalence of inflammatory disease in this country. In this chapter, we will return to those statistics and examine some of the major shifts in the world's food supply that may be responsible.

But when researchers and doctors are dealing with "the big picture," as we will be doing in this chapter, they sometimes have to remind themselves that these numbers aren't just numbers. They represent real people—people in danger, and people in pain. The statistics we'll be discussing represent our mothers, uncles, brothers, wives, and, perhaps most terrifyingly, our children.

Why Us?

We are unquestionably facing an epidemic in inflammatory disease. By my estimate, approximately half of all Americans suffer from an inflammatory disorder, and even more of us are at risk.

The central mystery behind this "epidemic of epidemics," including diseases like arthritis, asthma, allergies, lupus, and diabetes, is *why* it is happening. After all, it comes when American medicine and hygiene is unsurpassed. We've eliminated (or markedly reduced) many of the infectious diseases that shortened our life spans in the previous century. Smallpox, typhus, polio, cholera, and the bubonic plague are now the stuff of historical novels. The number of cases of (and fatalities from) the major killers of the early 1900s—like tuberculosis, polio, typhoid, whooping cough, and pneumonia—has fallen to fewer than fifty for every hundred thousand people. Over the past hundred years, the infant mortality rate in this country has decreased by a power of ten.

By contrast, noninfectious inflammatory diseases have gotten *worse* in each of the last three decades. A physician friend of mine jokes that Celebrex has replaced Prozac as the "must-have" drug of the decade. Doesn't it seem as if everyone you know is developing arthritis, allergies, or asthma? In the face of the tremendous success we have had in beating back conditions that no one thought we could ever conquer, inflammatory disease is besting us.

In fact, there's a shocking and counterintuitive surprise in the epidemiological evidence: the *more* developed the country, the *worse* the inflammatory epidemic. The best evidence for this statement comes from a study done by the International Study of Asthma and Allergy in Childhood (ISAAC), which sought to identify factors that might explain the rise in allergic diseases, a particularly pervasive inflammatory disorder. The study was massive, with over a half a million children aged six to seven and thirteen to fourteen years, from 155 medical centers, in fifty-six countries.

The ISAAC study showed that the highest prevalence of asthma symptoms was found mainly in affluent, English-speaking countries, like the United Kingdom and Australia. Symptoms were lowest in Eastern Europe, Russia, China, India, and Ethiopia. Identical trends were observed for hay fever and eczema.

> Ironically, something about our high standard of living is driving this epidemic of inflammatory diseases. Our affluence isn't alleviating our symptoms, it's making them worse!

So the sophisticated standard of living that so enhances the quality of our lives appears to correlate with the inflammation epidemic.

"I Don't *Feel* Affluent!"

You're probably thinking, Hey, I'm not affluent! None of us feel that we are, especially at the end of the month when the credit card bills arrive.

So what do I mean by affluence? In this instance, affluence isn't a personal characteristic, but a national one. It's countries we're talking about, not individuals. Compared to other countries, America is very rich and very developed. For instance, meat in this country is readily available practically everywhere, and it is relatively inexpensive. In fact, fresh fruits and vegetables are more expensive in some areas than a fast-food burger or fried chicken dinner. By contrast, a rural rice farmer in China is more likely to depend on his own garden and the garden of his neighbors for dinner, with meat as an only occasional addition. The more developed and industrialized the country, the more inflammatory disease there appears to be, which makes inflammation "a disease of affluence." Ironically, within affluent countries, it is often most painfully felt in some of the least affluent populations. For example, according to a study done by the Harlem Children's Zone Asthma Initiative in 2003, one out of every *four* children has asthma in central Harlem, one of New York City's poorest neighborhoods. That number is one of the highest ever documented in an American neighborhood, and fully twice what researchers expected to find when they began collecting data.

Theories to Explain the Pandemic of Inflammatory Diseases

In this book, I put forth a possible cause for this epidemic, but to be fair, my theory is not the only one. Many have been proposed, and some hold more water in my opinion than others. Consider the evidence for yourself:

The Gene Theory

One of the theories that has been put forth to explain this spike in inflammatory disease is genetic susceptibility: people in affluent countries share genes that predispose them to diseases like arthritis, asthma, heart disease, and diabetes.

There's no doubt that certain people are more genetically susceptible to these diseases than others. We know this because so many of these diseases run in families. But genes definitely aren't the only factor determining whether you have, or will get, one of these inflammatory conditions.

We know this because epidemiologists, people who study the factors affecting the distribution of diseases, tell us that even genetically similar people can have dramatically different levels of inflammation, depending on where they live.

Consider this. Children from Pakistan are *ten times* more likely to develop type 1 diabetes after moving to the United Kingdom than children who remain in Pakistan. In other words, just the move from a developing country to an industrialized nation increases these children's risk of diabetes tenfold. In another example, epidemiologists have determined that African Americans are much more likely to develop lupus than their genetically similar counterparts from the African continent. The difference, in both examples, is that the United Kingdom and the United States are fully industrialized; Pakistan and Africa are not.

Perhaps most striking are the epidemiological statistics after German unification. Germany was a single country, divided for a generation by a wall, which meant that the populations on either side of the wall were practically identical from a genetic point of view. The differences were in the cultures and in their wealth. West Germany enjoyed a booming economy and one of the highest standards of living in the world, including an annual per capita income that surpassed that of the United States, while East Germany struggled with poverty, a drastically lower standard of living, and comparatively poor health care.

How, then, to explain why children and adults in the poorer and less-developed East Germany suffered from fewer cases of asthma, allergy, and hay fever than children in the much more affluent West? Several comparative studies were done examining both children and adults in Sweden and Poland; Sweden and Estonia; Finland and Russia; the Baltic area; and Sweden, the Baltic countries, and Uzbekistan; and similar results were seen. The epidemiological evidence is clear: even in genetically similar populations, in extremely close geographic proximity, there is more inflammatory disease in more industrialized and affluent societies.

So it's not just our genes that are driving this disease. Something in our environment is making us sick.

The Pollution Theory

Invariably, one of the first ideas that people throw into the ring when I talk about the skyrocketing increase in asthma sufferers is the idea that the increase in asthma and allergies has to do with an increase in air pollution in industrialized countries. Even if this theory were correct, it wouldn't explain the dramatic increase in other inflammatory diseases like Crohn's disease and eczema. But let's examine the theory on its own merits.

Here's a shocker: air quality *hasn't* gotten worse. In fact, it's gotten significantly better—while the incidence of asthma has doubled in the last two decades. Air pollution in both the United States and Japan has improved drastically in the last twenty years, and yet asthma cases in both countries continue to rise steadily.

In fact, there doesn't seem to be much of a connection between air quality and inflammatory disease at all. In 2004, the Asthma and Allergy Foundation of America published a list that ranked the worst cities for people with asthma. The cities were judged according to fifteen factors, including the prevalence of the disease, the number of deaths it caused, the number of prescriptions filled, and the number of asthma specialists it was able to support.

Do you know which city ranked as the worst for asthma sufferers in the United States? If your first guess is a smog-filled urban center like New York, Washington, D.C., or Los Angeles—you're wrong. The worst city in the United States for asthma is Knoxville, Tennessee; it's followed by Little Rock, Arkansas, and St. Louis, Missouri. Where will you find bucolic Madison, Wisconsin? Also in the top ten worst cities—joined by Louisville, Kentucky, and Toledo, Ohio.

And what about all those big, filthy metropolises so notorious for their poor air quality? In fact, most of them ranked in the bottom half of the list. Atlanta came in at 47, Washington, D.C., at 50, Chicago at 56, and Los Angeles at 85. New York shared the number 32 spot with Scranton, Pennsylvania, while San Francisco and Miami topped the list as the *best* places to live.

Again, post-unification Germany provides us with an argument against the theory that pollution is the problem behind skyrocketing asthma. One of the top priorities after the Berlin wall came down was to do something about the dire situation the environment had gotten into while East Germany was cordoned off, economically and politically, from the world. The water was toxic, and, by some accounts, the air pollution was twice what would be tolerated in the United States. And yet, East German children living with pollution deemed worse than their neighboring countries suffered fewer instances of asthma.

So, although there are many, many good reasons to focus on cleaning up the quality of our air and water, pollution is probably not a major culprit behind the recent spike in this particular inflammatory disease.

The "Disease of Old Age" Theory

Still others have discounted the rise in inflammatory diseases, claiming that the increase is linked to our longer life expectancy. Let's look at this theory a little more closely. It's true that in the last century, before we'd advanced the war against infectious diseases like tuberculosis and pneumonia, people didn't live long enough to get "diseases of old age," like arthritis. Are modern medicine and our increased standard of living keeping people alive just so they can be felled by inflammatory diseases masquerading as diseases of old age?

Certainly, there are changes that take place in our bodies as we age that place us at higher risk of getting certain inflammatory diseases. And I will go into more detail in chapter 5 about why this is the case. But here again, the "old age" theory is weakened by the epidemiological evidence. Nearly 65 percent of people with arthritis are under sixty-five. We're *twice* as likely to develop this disease as our parents were, and at much younger ages. Most of the increase in inflammatory diseases has occurred at a time (from 1970 to the present) during which life spans have *not* significantly increased.

The insistence on seeing these inflammatory diseases as diseases of the elderly isn't just incorrect, but risky. When we calm ourselves with the false assurance that these are diseases of old age, it leaves us with a blind spot precisely where our concern should be most concentrated:

Children make up a large proportion of the new cases of these diseases—*not* the elderly.

If you have kids, you don't need to see statistics demonstrating the increase in these diseases; you'll know immediately what I'm talking about. Doesn't it seem as if more and more children have more serious allergies today than they did when we were kids? There was peanut-butter-cream icing on the chocolate cupcakes at my sixth birthday party—two great tastes that went great together. Now, nut allergies have become some of the most common and potentially deadly allergies, to the point at which airlines have replaced their traditional peanut snacks with pretzels and many schools don't allow children to bring their own snacks, lest they contain an allergen that might prove fatal for a classmate. And allergies aren't the only growing problem; you will likely see a lot more asthma inhalers at a sixth birthday party today than you did at mine in 1963. According to the Asthma and Allergy Foundation of America, the death rate for children nineteen years and younger from asthma increased by 78 percent between 1980 and 1993.

> One of the significant populations likely to be affected by inflammatory disease isn't older people, it's *our children.*

The Hygiene Hypothesis

In addition, others have put forth the hygiene hypothesis. The hygiene hypothesis is essentially the pollution theory turned inside out: it's not because we're dirty that we're getting sick, it's because we're too clean.

This theory suggests that increased cleanliness and a rise in the use of antibiotics in developed countries have inadvertently contributed to the allergy epidemic. Our houses are cleaner, our sewage is disposed of sanitarily, and our water supply is safer—with the result that our children are less exposed to disease-causing bacteria, infectious agents, and their by-products when they're very young. According to the theory, this has altered the way our immune system responds to harmless intruders. Proponents of the hygiene hypothesis say that because we're so clean and disease-free in childhood, our immune systems don't have the chance to develop normally through exposure to a wide variety of germs, and so they remain out of balance.

Several pivotal studies have examined this theory in children living in developed nations. Children who live on farms have a significantly lower prevalence of allergies than children from the same areas who don't live on farms. Complex statistical analysis identified these children's exposure to livestock and poultry as the feature of farm life that most protected them against asthma and hay fever.

Other studies have examined the role of infections on allergic diseases. Many of these studies show that the more infections young children have, the lower the likelihood that they will develop asthma and allergy. And the more siblings they have (carrying even more infectious agents), the better.

Although there is substantial evidence to support this theory, there are weaknesses to it as well. According to the hygiene hypothesis, one would expect that a wide variety of infections would *protect* against allergic diseases such as asthma, but, in fact, many infectious agents actually trigger allergic reactions and asthma symptoms. In many cases, infectious agents such as measles and respiratory viruses (especially ones in the lower respiratory tract) increase, rather than decrease, allergic diseases such as asthma. So although the hygiene hypothesis is a very promising theory that warrants further development, it doesn't fully apply to the whole scope of inflammatory diseases, including arthritis and diabetes.

Eating Ourselves Sick

So what's behind this epidemic? What change in our lifestyles can explain this explosion in inflammatory disease?

I believe that our diet is a major—if not the most important—external factor behind the inflammation epidemic.

Researchers have been trying to identify a dietary reason for inflammatory diseases for years, but like the proverbial blind men feeling their way around an elephant, they had only been able to identify parts of the puzzle. Strict vegetarian diets, for instance, have been studied for their effects on rheumatoid arthritis, but most of these studies lacked rigor, and the clinical improvement was minor. Other researchers have looked at food additives to see if there's a connection between them and

In fact, the cause of this inflammation pandemic may be right in front of us—flanked by a knife and fork.

some inflammatory diseases. Certain of the substances added to our food during processing, including monosodium glutamate, aspartame, various food dyes, and preservatives, are responsible for allergic reactions, including asthma, in some people. Some people may indeed be allergic to those additives, but not enough to explain an epidemic of inflammatory disease.

It's certainly no secret that the way we eat is out of sync with our body's needs. Most of the evolutionary forces that shaped our genetic development were exerted over ten thousand years ago when we were hunter-gatherers. Nothing in that programming could have prepared us for the Big Mac. Our bodies, and more specifically our genetics, simply aren't designed to eat the "foods of affluence" available to a twentieth-century urban dweller.

It is this disconnect that I blame for many of our current medical ills.

The Obesity Connection

This disconnect is also to blame for skyrocketing obesity rates—another public health issue that has grown to epidemic proportions over the last thirty years. According to the most recent statistics, published in the June 2004 edition of the *Journal of the American Medical Association (JAMA)*, 64 percent of American adults are overweight or obese. Sixteen percent of children are overweight, and 31 percent of those remaining are estimated to be at risk for overweight or obesity.

Inflammatory disease and obesity are not simply maladies running on parallel tracks, but are intrinsically intertwined for a number of reasons. There are a number of straightforward connections between those excess pounds and inflammatory disease.

One of these commonalities is what I call "foods of affluence," and the overwhelming quantities of some of those foods in the typical Western diet. For instance, early humans obtained more than half of their calories from carbohydrates, but most of these carbohydrates came from vegetables and fruit, with a smattering of beans and whole grains thrown in. In affluent societies, carbohydrates take the form of refined, added sugars and highly processed grain flours, highly caloric foods that provide us with none of the nutrients necessary for optimal health. The ready availability of eggs, meat, and poultry is another function of our affluence.

That's not the only connection. In fact, I believe that *obesity is one of the major driving forces behind inflammatory disease.* Fat cells themselves produce the inflammatory messengers that cause inflammatory disease. The more fat cells you have, and the bigger those cells are, the more inflammatory messengers you will produce, increasing the likelihood that you will have an inflammatory disease. Certainly much has been written about the very strong correlation between overweight and disease. Obesity has a direct impact on heart disease, diabetes, stroke, high blood pressure, some cancers, gout, osteoarthritis, and polycystic ovarian syndrome (PCOS). It's not an accident that you see quite a few diseases that fit into the category of inflammatory disease on that list. In fact, the correlation between fat and inflammation is explicit and direct. Inflammatory and obesity epidemics not only share a cause, but they play off each other, to our tremendous detriment. These conditions cannot often be separated. Obesity is an inflammatory condition, and being overweight makes inflammatory disease more severe. We cannot address one without addressing the other, and we cannot address either without changing what we eat.

> Being overweight increases the likelihood that you'll develop inflammatory disease, and it can make the inflammatory disease you have worse.

Planes, Trains, and Automobiles

To strike back effectively against the forces behind our Inflammation Nation, we should look at the global changes that have taken place, both in our dietary habits and in our food supply. I believe that those changes have caused a vast divide between the foods our bodies are designed to eat and what we're actually eating. This chasm may be one of the major keys to solving the mystery behind the inflammatory epidemic.

In 1800, the great majority (about 97 percent) of the world's populations lived in rural areas. By the year 2000, almost 76 percent of the inhabitants of developed countries lived in an urban environment. One of the results of this population shift has been unprecedented growth in—

and a significant change in the nutrient content of—the world's livestock industry.

In less-industrialized countries, people eat a lot of unprocessed grains and nonmeat proteins (like beans and soy) because they are both less expensive than meat, and because it's hard to store perishables when refrigeration is a luxury. Think, for instance, of a typical Asian meal, which consists of a wealth of rice and vegetables with a little meat added for variety and flavor. Compare that to a typical American plate, where meat, potatoes, and bread crowd out the vegetables—and dessert is an inevitability, not a treat.

Cities have an infrastructure to support the distribution of perishables like milk, eggs, meat, fish, and poultry before they spoil. All this has made meat comparatively plentiful—and inexpensive. It's now more expensive to prepare meals exclusively from fresh fruits, vegetables, and legumes! And meat is often inexpensive from a time standpoint as well. It's a lot easier—and a lot cheaper—to stop off at a fast-food place to pick up burgers or fried chicken with a side of fries or coleslaw for dinner than to shop for something to prepare. The drive-through is the problem!

This change in our diet has had a massive impact on food production in this country. In the last thirty years, as the world has become more industrialized, livestock consumption has increased a staggering 50 percent.

What About Fish?

Another major shift in our food supply is in the amount—and the *source*—of the fish we eat.

Humans used to eat more fish. In general, dietary consumption of fish has declined. This may have something to do with a shift in pricing; in most cases, it's cheaper to feed your family chicken, turkey, or pork than fresh fish. Fish is an important source of essential fatty acids, fatty acids that we cannot produce on our own. These fatty acids have tremendous impact on our health, with the result that the medical community is aggressively campaigning to get people to eat more fatty fish. The American Heart Association currently recommends that people without documented heart disease eat fish at least twice a week, and that people with documented heart disease eat fish every day.

I believe that these so-called "heart-healthy" recommendations may actually be contributing to making us very sick.

How?

Before answering that, I would like to stress one thing: the evidence is absolutely clear that long-chain omega-3 fatty acids from wild fish or fish-oil supplements—the "essential fatty acids"—*do* reduce the risk of heart attack and other problems related to heart and blood vessel disease. These fatty acids do not appear to alter total cholesterol, HDL cholesterol, or LDL cholesterol, but they can reduce triglycerides, high concentrations of which have been shown to be an important predictor of heart disease. I am amazed that people with heart disease in the United States take such limited advantage of this incredibly simple and safe solution to our nation's most devastating health problem.

But something has happened to make some fish a much less healthy food choice than we think it is. There has been a radical shift in where we get the fish we eat, a shift that has dramatic implications for our health. Wild fish reserves became seriously depleted by the 1970s for a number of reasons, ranging from the overfishing of our waters, to pollution, to dams and industrial development that interfered with the natural ability of fish to breed. This depletion led to an increase in aquaculture, or fish farming. This industry stepped in to address a serious deficit, and now, a large proportion of the fish eaten in developed countries is farmed.

I believe it's precisely these dietary shifts that lead us to some of the major culprits behind the inflammatory epidemic. We're designed to eat a certain balance of components in our diet. When you change that balance of components, it alters important metabolic events, which directly affect the way your body performs. Think of this another way: a high-end athlete burns enough calories to eat anything he wants to. Why, then, don't you see these high-performance athletes chowing down on deep-fried junk at fast-food joints? In fact, a professional athlete concentrates even more intensely on his food choices than the rest of us, because he understands that in order to coax the best performance out of his body, he has to encourage it with the best fuel.

The same thing is true for all of us. We also need a certain balance of these components to perform optimally, a balance we used to get without thinking about our diets. Now, we're no longer getting that balance because of the changes in the way our food is produced and the quantities in which we eat certain foods. I believe the resulting imbalance has adversely affected our health—fueling our inflammatory systems, which then remain on inappropriately high alert.

Over the course of this book, I hope to demonstrate that you can regain the balance lost by these changes in our food supply and content, simply by changing what you eat. Then, the food you eat will be working to improve your health, instead of fueling your inflammatory disease.

Chapter Two

The War Within

A security breach has been detected.

A deafening alarm goes up. Reconnaissance agents at the scene of the breach respond instantly and with military precision, sparking a series of maneuvers in lightning-quick succession. The precise nature of the intruder is assessed and decoded; target sets are defined; coordinates are mapped and synchronized. A lethal counterattack begins. Advance guerrilla troops move into location to mark and neutralize the invaders. On their intelligence, specialized commando troops are deployed, and wave after wave of lethal firepower rains down upon the interlopers.

When the firefight is over, the devastation is impressive. The still-smoking battlefield is littered with casualties from both sides, and the surrounding area is scorched and damaged. Cleanup crews arrive to carry away the dead and to extinguish any fires still burning, but even as they work, it is clear that the aftermath of this battle will be felt on this site for a long time.

Shock and Awe

No, this isn't a dispatch from the front lines of a war waged abroad; it's a representation of the complex sequence of events that happens when your body is called upon to defend itself—when you stub your toe, for instance, or start to come down with a cold. Your body has its own defense system—part of the immune system—and part of its arsenal is this process, which is called inflammation.

Since inflammation is at the root of a whole host of diseases plaguing our country, it is tempting to see the body's inflammatory response as the enemy, but this would be a terrible mistake. Indeed, this is part of the paradox behind inflammatory disease: there's nothing inherently wrong with inflammation; in fact, just the opposite is true.

The immune system's impressive show of inflammatory firepower is not only appropriate, but absolutely vital to sustaining life. It's not over-stating the case to say that inflammation is a keystone of your own health, and of our very survival as a species.

When your body is invaded by a virus or bacteria, it is your immune system that allows you to conquer that enemy. If your immune response is suppressed or underperforming, your body is left helpless and in danger. This is why people with immune deficiencies, like people living with AIDS (acquired immunodeficiency syndrome), are so vulnerable to op-portunistic infection that their immune systems can't respond to even the most pathetic challenger. And so, as we've seen all too often over the last twenty years, exposure to something as innocuous as the common cold can be fatal for someone with AIDS.

Your body's immune system is a complex and elegant one, designed to recognize and destroy any invader that has the potential to harm you. In this chapter, we'll explore how this highly sophisticated system works to protect the body when it's functioning normally.

Inflammation 101

First Lines of Defense

In the first place, your body has many layers of security in place to stop hostile intruders, before your immune system even gets involved. Skin, for instance, provides a barrier that keeps out a host of intruders. It also secretes various antibacterial agents that neutralize many bacteria on contact. Other likely entry sites, like your eyes, mouth, and nose, are lined with mucous membranes that catch and destroy potential invaders before they can get into your bloodstream.

The Surveillance Units

If an invader manages to penetrate these defenses and enter the blood-stream, specially designed surveillance cells set off an extremely sophisti-cated alarm system. These surveillance cells act as command and control centers for the attack against the invader; their alarms activate the body's immune system. An invader can be anything from bacteria, to a virus, to a parasite, to cancer cells.

The alarm system is exquisitely complex, with a number of component parts. The surveillance cells release their own on-site defenses, but they also send a variety of chemical messages throughout the body, asking for help and reinforcements. In response to these chemical messengers, your body sends out its army: ground troops in the form of white blood cells made in the marrow of our bones.

The Ground Troops

This white blood cell army is made up of different divisions, which perform specialized functions. One kind, called **B lymphocytes,** acts as the advance guard by making antibodies, which are specialized proteins designed to attack bacteria, viruses, and toxic proteins. Another type of white blood cell, called **neutrophils,** has a very short life span. They're ferociously destructive, designed to use the little time they have to maximum effect, so they act like kamikaze pilots or cluster bombs, taking out everything in their path. **Macrophages,** a third type of white blood cell, specialize in gobbling up the invaders and in releasing antibacterial enzymes that function much like a cleanup squad. Still another kind, called **T lymphocytes,** or T cells, tracks down and destroys invaders that have escaped the bloodstream and are hiding out in the tissues. These T cells either destroy the cells that have been altered by the invaders, or request reinforcements in the form of other, better-qualified types of white blood cells.

The Signalers: Inflammatory Messengers

At the site of the attack, the white blood cells and other tissue cells produce their own signals that aid in destroying the invader. One important weapon in the inflammatory chemical arsenal is the messengers of inflammation. A major family of inflammatory messengers is made up of complex fatty acids. These inflammatory messengers include molecules

called **leukotrienes** (pronounced loo-ko-try-eens) and **prostaglandins,**
which are made from a fatty acid called arachidonic
acid, or AA.

> **Leukotrienes and prostaglandins are central inflammatory messengers.**

These messengers play a crucial role in the inflammatory process, and we will return to them
again and again over the course of this book. Un-
surprisingly, these inflammatory messengers are responsible for many of the signs and symptoms we
traditionally associate with inflammation.

Prostaglandins

When you get a paper cut, the area swells and reddens, and the surrounding tissue is sensitive to the touch. Prostaglandins are to blame, and here's
why. These messengers encourage the blood vessels in the area around the
insult to dilate, so that it's easier for the white blood cell army to get
where it needs to go. The blood rushing out of the vessels manifests itself
in swelling and redness, two of the key indicators of inflammation.

Additionally, prostaglandins stimulate nerves that send pain messages
to the brain. Pain is a message in its own right: it tells you to stop what
you're doing, in case what you're doing is causing the pain. Without pain,

> **Blocking the production of prostaglandins short-circuits the pain associated with inflammation.**

you wouldn't know to take your hand off the hot ket-
tle. Without pain, you might jog on that sore knee
before it healed completely. So, on the off chance
that something you're doing is causing the inflammatory response, prostaglandins and other inflammatory messengers send up the pain alarm.

Many over-the-counter pain relievers, like aspirin
and ibuprofen, are designed to block the production of prostaglandins.

Leukotrienes

Leukotrienes, another type of inflammatory messenger in this family,
help direct the white blood cell army. These messengers call for troops,
and when those troops arrive, it's the leukotrienes that tell them where to
go—and how many battalions to send. Ideally, the attack the body
launches against the invader must be sufficiently brutal to immobilize

the enemy, but controlled enough so that the attack doesn't destroy the cells and tissues surrounding the battlefield. The amount of leukotrienes present at the scene of the white blood cells' attack influences the *scale* of that attack.

> The scale of the attack is determined by the number of the leukotrienes present at the scene.

Once the white blood cells have entered the tissues, the leukotrienes assume a supporting, but nonetheless important, role. They get the white blood cells ready to release their weapons array, and they keep those white blood cell soldiers alive for much longer than they'd be able to survive on their own.

So there's a wide variety of highly specialized troops doing battle in our bodies when security is breached, all masterminded and controlled by the inflammatory messengers. For the record, there are many types of inflammatory messengers, but prostaglandins and leukotrienes are the central players in a critical pathway that causes pain and inflammation, and can be controlled through diet. So we will be focusing on them for the purposes of this book. Reducing the production of these inflammatory messengers is the key way the Chilton Program is so effective in curbing overactive inflammation.

The Battle Site: The Body's Tissue

When the immune system launches a blitzkrieg like the one described at the beginning of this chapter, the surrounding tissues are destroyed. Ordinarily, the tissues repair themselves in the normal course of healing, and life goes on—a little reparable tissue damage is a small price to pay for a successfully vanquished infection.

But it's here, on the battle site of the body's tissues, that the worst damage is done when the normal inflammatory process becomes abnormal.

How Inflammation Becomes Disease

If you suffer from a chronic inflammatory disease (or love someone who does), you're all too aware that the vital process of inflammation—so essential to our continued health and well-being—can also be the engine of a tremendous deal of pain and suffering.

So where is the disconnect? How can something so central and important to our good health go so terribly wrong, and why does a process so essential to our survival as a species now threaten us in such epidemic numbers?

Too Much of a Good Thing

Inflammatory disease is, simply put, too much of a good thing. The inflammatory process operates in fundamentally the same way whether your body is attacking a legitimate target, like an infection, or attacking itself, as it does when you have inflammatory disease.

> Inflammatory disease is just an exaggeration of the normal immune system response.

We're used to thinking of disease as what happens when some vital organ or system in the body stops working—if your eyes don't work, you can't see. By contrast, inflammatory disease isn't caused by a malfunction in the way the system works. The system, in fact,

The War Within
Phase I: On the Brink of War

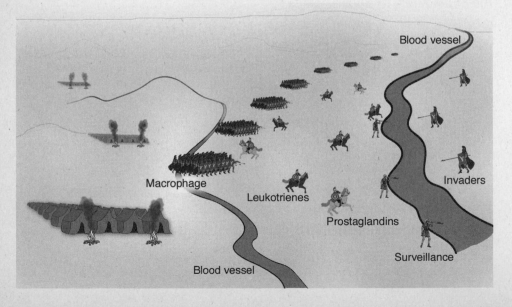

Blood vessel

Macrophage

Leukotrienes

Prostaglandins

Invaders

Surveillance

Blood vessel

The War Within

Phase II: The Battle in the Tissues

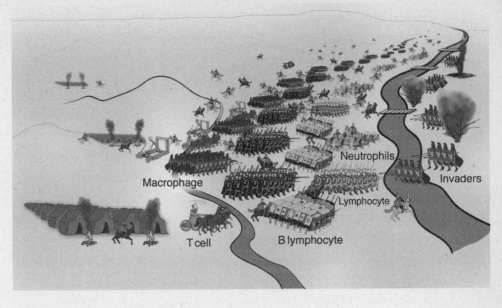

The War Within

Phase III: The Devastation of War

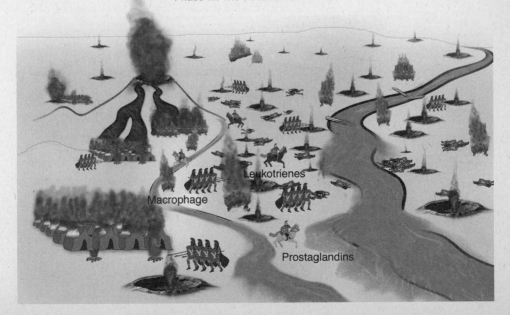

is perfectly okay—it's just firing too frequently. The internal dial in our bodies, set to trigger this essential defense reaction, is permanently set on "red alert."

Inflammatory disease is, in practice, the opposite of AIDS and other immunodeficiency disorders. In those diseases, the security guard is asleep at the desk. Arthritis, asthma, and other inflammatory diseases are what happens when that pendulum swings the other way.

More Messengers, More Problems

Clearly, inflammation, even when it's occurring appropriately, leaves its mark. The outsized amplification of that system in a person with inflammatory disease just increases the devastation.

As we now know, inflammatory disease begins with a miscalculation. The body believes it's defending itself, but in reality, it's waging war against either a harmless bystander, or, worse, against its own healthy tissues. The intelligence failure doesn't stop there. The body is not only requesting troops in error, but as part of the overreaction it sends too many messengers, with an abundance of requests. It's like hitting the button on the photocopier a hundred times when you need only one copy.

The system is flooded with these messengers—and given what you now know about the way those messengers work, you can see why inflammatory diseases are so painful and so destructive.

> When you have an inflammatory disease, the body produces too many of those inflammatory messengers, leukotrienes and prostaglandins.

The more prostaglandins the body produces, the more the blood vessels will dilate, which translates into more redness and swelling. More prostaglandins also means more pain. More leukotrienes, on the other hand, means the body dispatches even more white blood cells, which in turn do even *more* damage to the tissue. And the more leukotrienes you have, the longer those white blood cells are able to stay alive, doing more damage to the surrounding battlefield.

When Healing Hurts

The body weathers a tremendous amount of damage when you have an inflammatory disease. There's always tissue damage associated with inflammation, even when the target is an appropriate one, like bacteria or an infection. Your body also has a tremendous capacity to repair itself, and under ordinary circumstances, the body repairs itself quite well. Unfortunately, when you have chronic inflammatory disease, the toll rises much, much higher. Because there are too many messengers, the whole firefight—often misguided from its very inception—is happening on an enormous scale. And the chronic nature of inflammatory disease means that it's happening over, and over, and over again.

Battalion after battalion of white blood cells floods the area where the harmless invader has been detected, and the injury to the adjacent tissues is ruinous. It's like using a blowtorch to light the candles on a birthday cake. The body's cleanup efforts only compound the damage. When this kind of heavy-duty tissue damage is taking place on an unremitting and persistent basis, as it is when you have an inflammatory disease, your body never has the time to catch up on healing. Instead, you're trapped in an endless and ultimately destructive cycle of damage and partial repair, damage and partial repair—a relentless feedback loop that scorches the battlefield, leaving you exhausted and often resulting in chronic pain.

> Inflammatory disease is chronic—both long-lasting and recurrent—so the body can't ever completely heal.

Eventually, the steady struggle within the tissue begins to disrupt the basic structure and function of the battlefield itself. The repeated assaults and partial repairs leave tissue that is permanently damaged and scarred. A scar on the skin is usually nothing more than an unsightly aberration. A scar on the organs and tissues *inside* the body can be a bigger problem. The scars that result from the chronic warfare taking place in the joints of someone living with rheumatoid arthritis may eventually warp and distort the joint itself, rendering it unable to work the way it was designed to work. It is scarring that causes intestinal obstruction in people who suffer from Crohn's disease, and arterial scarring that causes atherosclerosis.

Acute and Chronic Insults

In many diseases, inflammation is acute, which means that the condition has a sudden onset and will run a short course. As we've seen, the destruction that accompanies acute inflammation is destruction the body can cope with and heal—as long as it eventually ends. The difference between an acute and a chronic inflammatory disease is the length of time the inflammatory response is permitted to damage the tissues.

So, for instance, you might be surprised to find bronchitis on a list of inflammatory diseases, because you think of it simply as the bad cough you got after a particularly bad head cold, the one that went away quickly after your doctor gave you antibiotics. That *is* bronchitis, but of the acute variety. Acute bronchitis *is* an inflammatory condition, but in this case, inflammation is doing the job it's supposed to do—rallying to defend your system against an insult to the lungs.

Chronic inflammation is the result of chronic insult. So, chronic bronchitis is what happens when the insult to your lungs is repeated over and over again. Inflammation has to take up permanent residence to defend your body against a threat it can never fully rebuff. Cigarette smoking, one of the leading causes of chronic bronchitis, is just such a repeated insult. A chronic cigarette habit means that your body requires full-time security to "protect" your lungs against the toxins attacking them; eventually, that chronic inflammation will scar your lungs.

The Noises in the Dark

When you have an inflammatory disease, your immune system is set on a hair trigger, poised to react even when the "invaders" in question are actually harmless—a dust particle, animal dander, pollen.

If the normal inflammatory process is a measured tactical response to an accurately perceived threat, then chronic inflammatory disease is a loose cannon, both gun-happy and paranoid, shooting indiscriminately at every sound in the darkness.

In fact, there are different types of "noises in the dark" that trigger this type of overheated response from the immune system in someone who has inflammatory disease. There is the category of inflammatory disease called allergic disease. The body's own cells may also trigger this kind of overresponse; those diseases are called autoimmune diseases. Several inflammatory diseases occur in people who are also overweight, causing scientists to examine whether obesity can be implicated in the inception of the inflammatory response. And there are many diseases for which we simply do not yet know what the trigger is.

The Allergic Overreaction

Allergy is the smoking gun behind many inflammatory diseases, including allergies, asthma, and many skin diseases. An allergic reaction happens when your body's immune system becomes so hypersensitive that it breaks out the big guns in response to the most harmless invader. A dust particle poses no real threat to most healthy individuals, but if you're someone who's sensitive to this allergen, your body perceives this innocuous interloper as a serious threat, and responds accordingly.

The body's reaction to the perceived threat is the real danger behind allergies. Take the potentially lethal peanut allergy. In truth, it's not the peanut that hurts you, but your body's *overreaction* to that peanut: if you are someone who suffers from this very common (and very dangerous) allergy, the inflammatory overreaction in your lungs results in something called anaphylaxis; in other words, your airways close, making it difficult for you to breathe and get the oxygen you need to survive. The terrible irony, of course, is that many of these severe allergic reactions—to seemingly inoffensive substances like golden pollen dust or a nut—can be life-threatening in themselves.

Autoimmunity: Friendly Fire

Autoimmune disorders, like rheumatoid arthritis and lupus, make up another major category of chronic inflammatory disease. In these disorders, your body isn't overreacting to a harmless intruder, as it is with an allergy, but to itself. In effect, your body becomes allergic to its own tissues, responding to them as though they were hostile trespassers. Friendly fire is the metaphor that I most often use to describe these disorders, and it's an apt one. In every war, there are casualties. They are a terrible and heavy price to pay, but they are an understood cost. Not so when the causalities happen in error—the result of a bomb dropped, or weapons fired, on allies. It's every soldier's worst nightmare: an intelligence failure that lands him in an inadvertent firefight against his own side. This is precisely what happens in autoimmune diseases: the system in place to protect your body from infection and disease attacks the body itself. So when you're living with an autoimmune disease, friendly fire—and the fratricide associated with it—are a way of life.

How does such a blunder occur? The body's defense system is designed to defend against foreign threat. In order to do this effectively, it must reliably know how to distinguish "self" from "other"—a complicated and sophisticated calculation, and one that the body does automatically and with spectacular precision, as long as the immune system is functioning normally. Unfortunately, for reasons not yet completely understood, that recognition system can become unreliable.

> When you have an autoimmune disease, the body's defense system attacks *its own* cells and tissues as if they were invaders.

When the gatekeepers can no longer be trusted to distinguish between native and foreign, the body begins to launch campaigns against itself in a process called autoimmunity.

Obesity: Chicken—or Egg?

You've certainly noticed the overlap between what I call the twin epidemics of inflammation and obesity: many inflammatory diseases, like heart disease and diabetes, are also diseases associated with obesity. Being overweight increases the likelihood that you will be diagnosed with an inflammatory disease, and being overweight will likely exacerbate an inflammatory disease you already have. But is obesity the chicken—or the egg?

In fact, it's the chicken.

We now know that obesity is one of the primary driving forces behind the overactive inflammation that causes disease.

> Obesity *causes* inflammation.

That's why I've listed it here, along with other "causes" of an inappropriate immune response, like allergens or the body's failure to recognize its own tissues. How does being overweight trigger overactive inflammation? The search for an answer to this question is emerging as one of the hottest areas in scientific research today. Let's look at what we know.

While it may be tempting to think of fat simply as the stuff that hangs over your belt, it's a dangerous misperception. In the past few decades, scientists have discovered that fat is very active, metabolically. Fat cells are "large and in charge"—they direct a large number of the chemical interactions and processes that go into maintaining the body. In fact, the scientists who study fat think of it more as a gland or an organ, because of the way fat cells act as a control center for many of the processes that determine how our body behaves.

This is one of the reasons that obesity is now recognized as a chronic inflammatory state. One of the things your fat cells are doing (in addition to hanging over your belt) is making inflammatory messengers the same way white blood cells do when they react to your body being attacked.

There may have been an evolutionary reason for this. Fat cells, in addition to having a critical role in fat metabolism, play an important role in supplementing the immune systems of several members of the animal kingdom, including humans. According to G. S. Hotamisligil, people whose fat cells had developed inflammatory pathways would have had a better chance of surviving infectious diseases—probably the biggest threat to life at that point in evolution—so natural selection favored those pathways. Now, our early ancestors lived in much less abundant times, and would never have gotten enough calories for those fat cells to become metabolically overactive, or for the inflammatory pathways they produced to get out of control. We, on the other hand, get more than enough, with disastrous consequences for our immune systems.

The fatter we get, the worse it becomes. Most of the time, you don't make more fat cells when you gain weight; the ones you have just get fatter. But when those cells have gotten as big as they can get, you do create more cells. Overweight people have bigger fat cells, and very overweight people have more of them. Research has shown that large fat cells *do* more—are more metabolically active—than their smaller counterparts. So when the fat cells are making inflammatory messengers in an overweight person, they're making an abnormally large amount of those messengers, which is thought to be the key mechanism by which obesity affects inflammatory disease.

It gets worse! In general, overweight people make more of everything, but there's an important exception: overweight people make *less* of a hormone called adiponectin. If you're at a normal weight, adiponectin is circulating at a relatively high concentration in your blood; those levels drop precipitously when you're overweight. That's really too bad, because adiponectin, which is exclusively produced by fat cells, has a number of potent anti-inflammatory properties. For instance, it inhibits the production of one of the pro-inflammatory messengers (TNF-alpha) made by fat cells.

So not only are the fat cells of the overweight making *more* inflammatory messengers, but they make *less* of one of the most powerful anti-inflammatory hormones.

Given that approximately a third of all Americans are considered to be overweight, we cannot ignore this inflammatory trigger.

Unknown Origin

In some cases, researchers have not yet put all the pieces of the puzzle together to discover why the chronic inflammation causing these diseases has taken up residence in the body's tissues. In some diseases, such as psoriasis and Crohn's disease, we know that a malfunction in the immune system is causing the inflammation that powers that particular disease, but we're not sure where the malfunction takes place, or what causes it. This can be very frustrating. It's very stressful and upsetting to learn that you have a disease—and that distress is often compounded when you realize that your doctor has no idea why your body has turned against itself in this way.

Even if your disease is one of the ones with a mystery behind its origin, please don't despair. While that information is certainly central to a full understanding of these diseases, it's actually secondary to our own purpose, which is to make you feel better and to improve your disease state by reducing inflammation. Even if we don't know the precise reason why your body is attacking itself, it's the inflammation that's causing the tissue damage. I believe that addressing the inflammation by following the Chilton Program will help your symptoms, no matter what dysfunction in the body is causing the initial misfire.

Inflammatory Disease: A Preexisting Condition?

As you've seen, it takes just a slight shift of the pendulum to move from an inflammatory system that's working normally to protect your body from harmful aggressors to an inflammatory system on overdrive. Inflammatory disease isn't an instance of a system failure, but of a system on inappropriately high alert. Your inflammatory system doesn't work differently when you have inflammatory disease, it just works *more*. The song is the same, but the volume is turned up way too high.

Anyone who's spent any time with a four-year-old is no stranger to what I call "the constant why." For a four-year-old, no answer is satisfactory—there's always another layer of the onion to be peeled back, with another "why?" waiting underneath. We don't know why inflammatory disease happens, and as a result it turns all of us—researchers, doctors, and patients alike—into four-year-olds, endlessly pursuing the constant why, with no satisfaction in sight.

> We don't know why inflammatory disease happens.

Aside from chronic insult, we don't know why certain people are struck down by inflammatory disease. "Why do I have allergies?" "Because your body overreacts to a harmless allergen." "Why?" "You seem to be genetically susceptible." "Why?" And eventually, the answers peter out, because we don't know why. But I suspect, based on twenty years of research, that it has a great deal to do with changes in our food supply. Since inflammatory disease is just an instance of a normal process on overdrive, this further explains why every single one of us is at risk, unless we make a course correction right now. Every one of us has this inflammatory capability, but for some of us, that pendulum has not yet begun its treacherous journey to the other side.

Because it's not the process of inflammation that changes with the onset of inflammatory disease, but simply the *amount*, can't we almost call inflammatory disease a preexisting condition, one that is likely to be triggered unless we act in order to get out of its path?

Yes, some of us are genetically predisposed to get these diseases—a great many of us, in fact. But there's no surefire way to tell in advance, no diagnostic test to alert you if you're in the line of fire. Researchers and epidemiologists are, in fact, seeing spikes in inflammatory disease in new populations, people who had not previously had a high incidence of those diseases. Among children, for instance, asthma has been growing at an astonishing rate.

It's terrifying. The changes that have brought us here are massive and global, and a hundred-plus years in the making, and they have left each one of us teetering on a precipice, so that this ordinary, life-saving process needs just the slightest nudge from us to morph into its darkest expression. What's worse, I believe we're tacitly giving that permission at every meal, with every mouthful we take.

That is why you'll find a Prevention Diet in this book. If you are one of the lucky ones who are not living with inflammatory disease, it's essential to do everything within your power to make sure that you keep that pendulum's swing under control.

If you *do* suffer from one of these diseases, the Chilton Solution will finally give you the tools you need to help bring your inflammatory system back into balance.

You now know what inflammation is, and how overactive inflammation turns into disease. You may now be wondering, What does this have to do with me? What role does inflammation *really* play in diseases like arthritis, allergies, heart disease, and asthma?

Inflammation is a component in many human diseases, even those we do not consider to be inflammatory—it's our body's central defense, and how we respond to *everything* the body interprets as a threat. The difference is in the role that inflammation plays. It is these questions that we will be examining in detail in this chapter.

Crossing the Border Between Good and Poor Health

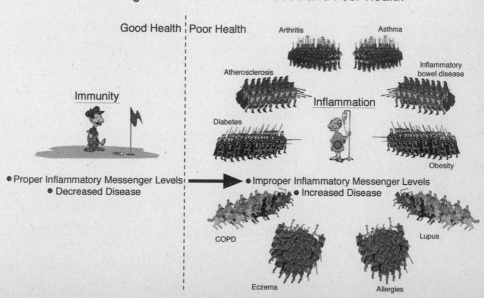

Good Health | Poor Health

Arthritis Asthma

Atherosclerosis Inflammatory
bowel disease

Immunity Inflammation

Diabetes

Obesity

● Proper Inflammatory Messenger Levels ● Improper Inflammatory Messenger Levels
● Decreased Disease ● Increased Disease

COPD Lupus

Eczema Allergies

The Three Categories of Inflammatory Disease

In fact, modern medicine is just beginning to understand the fundamental role the immune system and overactive inflammation play in many diseases that only a decade ago were thought not to involve inflammation—and we're finding inflammation and inflammatory messengers in places we never expected.

Recently, three of my colleagues and I met to design the Inflammatory Quotient quiz on page 141 of this book. There was a cardiologist, an infectious disease specialist, a clinical immunologist, and a molecular biologist at that table, each a recognized expert in his field.

The question I asked was this: which human diseases have an inflammatory component? I would like to note that the three categories we arrived at are based on our current state of knowledge, which means that they are fluid and changing, as research progresses. (Stay tuned, there will be more on this shifting paradigm later in the chapter.)

These were the three categories we came to:

◆ diseases *known* to be caused by overactive inflammation
◆ diseases *thought* to be caused by overactive inflammation
◆ diseases in which overactive inflammation *is suspected*

> There is much to be gained from bringing overactive inflammation back into balance— whether inflammation is the primary driving force, or takes only a supporting role.

I would strongly argue that there is much to be gained from bringing overactive inflammation back into balance, and in treating the inflammatory component of diseases—whether inflammation is the primary driving force of those diseases, or takes only a supporting role.

Let us now look at some examples of diseases in each category.

Diseases Known to Be Caused by Inflammation

The information we have tells us that inflammation is the primary cause of these diseases. In other words, an overwhelming number of clinical studies indicate that bringing inflammation back into balance will signif-icantly alleviate the symptoms of these diseases in the vast majority of sufferers.

Asthma

Asthma is the classic example of a disease in which inflammation is the primary driving force. It is a disease in which the airways, or passages of the lungs, become inflamed and swollen, making it difficult to breathe. Symptoms include wheezing, coughing, a sensation of tightness in the chest and throat, and an inability to take a deep, satisfying breath.

The most common form of asthma—estimated to be 60 percent of cases—is allergic asthma, which is triggered when you inhale or eat some-thing to which you're allergic. In this type of asthma, normally harmless substances, like pollen, trigger key "command and control" centers, which leads to the production of potent inflammatory messengers. These, in turn, mobilize battalions of white cells to the "battlefields" located in small airways, and their firefight causes structural damage to the lining of the airways, causing lung dysfunction. The pollen you inhale contains certain elements on its surface that the body recognizes as foreign. Once it has been marked by the body as a bad guy, it is rapidly recognized again the next time you inhale it, which leads to an asthma attack.

Twenty years ago when I begin to work on inflammatory messengers in airways, asthma was not categorized as an inflammatory disease. We simply thought it resulted from airways that were too small, or hypersen-sitive. Although both of these statements can be true about asthmatics, we now understand that inflammation is the root cause of this disease, and addressing and correcting that overactive inflammation became a primary treatment goal. For instance, understanding the role inflammation plays in asthma allowed researchers and pharmaceutical companies to develop a new generation of anti-inflammatory drugs—safer, more efficacious, and more easily tolerated—to prevent and manage attacks.

Allergies

By far the most common allergy is allergic rhinitis, known as "hay fever." Here, normally harmless substances, like pollen, trigger key "command

and control" centers to produce potent inflammatory messengers. These, in turn, mobilize battalions of white cells to the "battlefields" located, in this case, in the upper airways, and their firefight causes structural damage to the lining of the upper airways, causing sneezing and mucus secretion. Essentially, hay fever is allergic asthma of the nose.

Rheumatoid Arthritis

Rheumatoid arthritis (RA) is another form of inflammatory disease: instead of an allergic disease, caused by an external stimulus, RA occurs when the immune system attacks the body's own healthy tissue in the lining of the joints and other internal organs, causing inflammation.

Symptoms of this disease include general fatigue, as well as pain, swelling, stiffness, and warmth in the affected joints. Inflammatory cells can move into neighboring bone and cartilage, and release enzymes that eventually destroy that tissue. As the damage becomes permanent, the joint may lose its shape altogether, causing loss of function.

People who suffer from (or who, because of a family history or other factors, are at risk for) asthma, rheumatoid arthritis, and the other diseases in this category have much to gain from adopting an anti-inflammatory dietary strategy like the Chilton Program.

OTHER DISEASES KNOWN TO BE CAUSED BY OVERACTIVE INFLAMMATION

ATOPIC DERMATITIS is a skin inflammation that frequently accompanies allergies and asthma and often occurs among multiple members of a family. It usually appears as a reddish, swollen, itchy rash. If the rash results in open sores, you may be at risk for infection.

GOUT is an inflammatory disease of the joints, the result of crystalline uric acid deposits in the joints. In more than half of the people who develop gout, the inflammation first appears in the joint of the big toe.

LUPUS is a chronic inflammatory autoimmune disease; specialized proteins made by the body attack and destroy the body's own tissue. There is no diagnostic test for lupus. Symptoms of lupus include fatigue, muscle pain and weakness, a rash across the cheeks and nose, and fever and headaches; having lupus can make it difficult for a woman to carry a pregnancy to term.

INFLAMMATORY BOWEL DISEASE (IBD) is, as the name suggests, a category of diseases caused by a chronic inflammatory response in the large and small intestines. Within this larger category are a number of specific diseases. **Crohn's disease** tends to appear in the lower part of the small intestines, while **ulcerative colitis** is usually in the upper part of the large intestine, although both may appear anywhere in the digestive tract. Symptoms for both diseases include abdominal pain, cramping, fever, and diarrhea. Reduced appetite, weight loss, and even malnutrition may result. Scarring as a result of the inflammatory process may cause blockages in the intestines and narrowing of the digestive passageways; and both diseases may cause open sores, or ulcers, in the digestive system, which can become very serious. In people with **celiac disease (sprue),** eating gluten (found in wheat, barley, rye, and oats), sets off an immune response that causes damage to the small intestine, which then cannot absorb nutrients from food, resulting in malnutrition.

PSORIASIS is an inflammatory skin disease in which malfunctioning white cells send inflammatory messages to the skin cells, which make them reproduce and mature at an accelerated pace. Layers of dead cells accumulate on the surface of the skin, resulting in painful, dry, cracked, or blistered areas that often have silver flakes or scales on top. **Psoriatic arthritis,** a more serious form of the disease, occurs when psoriasis attacks the joints. Symptoms of psoriatic arthritis are similar to those of rheumatoid arthritis, including pain, stiffness, and swelling in the joints.

SCLERODERMA means "hard skin," and it is informally known as the disease that turns people into stone. An autoimmune disorder causes the overproduction of collagen, which causes the skin to harden. There are two kinds of scleroderma: localized, which is limited to the small areas of the skin, and diffuse, or systemic, which can affect large areas of the skin, the joints, and the internal organs.

Diseases *Thought* to Be Caused by Overactive Inflammation

In this category, the information we have about the role that inflammation plays in these diseases is less definitive. In most cases, there are convincing studies to indicate that inflammation is a component—and quite possibly the major component—of the disease. However, more conclusive clinical trials, specifically those that target inflammation's role, are essential to cement our understanding.

People with diseases in this category—and the cutting-edge physicians who treat them—often see a significant improvement in disease symptoms when they use anti-inflammatory therapies as part of their protocol.

Atherosclerosis

Atherosclerosis, a vascular disease caused by the hardening of the arteries, is responsible for the majority of cases of heart disease. Just as we were finally able to understand inflammation's role in asthma, a very similar paradigm shift is happening right now in cardiology.

Researchers used to think that buildup on the artery walls caused the arterial passageways to narrow, like a clogged drain, until blood could no longer get through, ultimately causing a heart attack. As a result, cardiologists had always considered atherosclerosis to be a lipid-storage disease, with cholesterol as the primary culprit.

Accumulating evidence now reveals that inflammation plays a key role in the development and progression of coronary artery disease. Inflammatory cells that live in the artery gobble up fats like cholesterol and triglycerides that accumulate there. If they eat enough of them, these inflammatory cells turn into foam cells (they look like foam). These foam cells have a relatively short life span, and when they die in the arteries, they explode, dumping their toxic foam baggage into the blood vessel, where it causes damage, and—you guessed it—more inflammation.

The cleanup crews call in muscle cells to form a protective cap over the rapidly accumulating mess. If the repair is incomplete, or the local tissue battlefield is too unstable, the cap can rupture, causing clots to form. These clots can completely block the inside of the artery, leading to a heart attack or stroke.

The evidence that atherosclerosis is an inflammatory disease has been significantly bolstered by studies that show the predictive power of a marker of inflammation called C-reactive protein (CRP). CRP is a blood protein that binds to bacterial walls, marking them for the body to recognize and destroy later. Inflammatory events that cause the production of inflammatory messengers stimulate the liver to produce CRP. CRP is usually low in normal individuals, but can rise one-hundred- to two-hundred-fold during acute inflammation.

CRP was discovered over seventy years ago, but cardiologists have more recently found that CRP can be a good predictor of a future heart attack or stroke in apparently healthy people. CRP is a particularly powerful predictor when it is combined with cholesterol measurements: when a person has high CRP and high cholesterol, they are *nine* times as likely to have a heart attack or stroke as people with low CRP and low cholesterol.

The inflammatory connection becomes even clearer when we look at atherosclerosis in the context of other inflammatory diseases. Indeed, the disease looks very much like rheumatoid arthritis, except that it occurs in the artery walls, and not the joints. Both diseases involve many of the same inflammatory cells and inflammatory messengers, and CRP is elevated in both.

The identification and treatment of inflammation as a serious contributor to heart disease, stroke, and many other chronic human diseases is one of the major shifts currently taking place in the scientific community. As they did with asthma twenty years ago, scientists and pharmaceutical companies are now looking to develop new anti-inflammatory drugs (and to utilize those medications currently available) to treat this disease, and others that now appear to have major inflammatory components.

Diabetes

Diabetes is a metabolic disorder, characterized by high blood glucose. The hormone that moves glucose into the cells so it can be used for energy is called insulin. Whenever you eat something, glucose is released into your bloodstream. Insulin picks up the glucose in the bloodstream and ferries it into cells where it's stored for further use. The amount of insulin your body releases increases (or decreases) depending on the demand. If there's a lot of sugar and fat in the bloodstream, you'll release a lot of insulin to carry it away.

The system works well, unless you regularly eat a lot of sugar, or eat too much in general. Then your body releases insulin constantly, in anticipation of your next rush. Eventually, like the townspeople with the little boy who cried wolf, your cells stop responding to the insulin.

This is a very dangerous state of affairs. If insulin isn't working, then blood sugar levels can get out of control very quickly. This situation is called insulin resistance, and is considered to be a pre-diabetic condition because it is the single biggest factor leading up to type 2 diabetes. It is estimated that by the year 2020, the number of people in the world with type 2 diabetes will grow to over 250 million people.

People with diabetes also have elevated levels of certain inflammatory messengers, which have been shown to cause insulin resistance, a primary symptom of diabetes. Anti-inflammatory medications have been proven to reduce the risk of developing both type 1 (early-onset) and type 2 (late-onset) diabetes.

OTHER DISEASES THOUGHT TO BE CAUSED BY OVERACTIVE INFLAMMATION

This category is for those diseases with a significant inflammatory component. They may, with more research and time, turn out to be inflammatory diseases, but at least for right now, there is an equal body of evidence supporting another cause.

CHRONIC KIDNEY FAILURE is often the result of mild but recurring inflammation which leads to the scarring that eventually reduces the efficiency of the kidneys in clearing waste products from the blood.

CHRONIC HEPATITIS (hepatitis means "inflammation of the liver") is caused when cells in the liver are damaged. The injury may be the result of alcohol abuse, drugs, disease, or an autoimmune disorder. The inflammation damages the liver, and the body's repair efforts result in scars, which cause **cirrhosis,** or irreversible scarring. This scarring makes it difficult for this essential organ to purify the blood and make essential nutrients.

CHRONIC THYROID DISEASE is most commonly caused by an autoimmune disorder, which causes the body to attack thyroid cells. Eventually enough of them are destroyed so that the gland can no longer produce hormones or regulate the metabolism effectively.

CHRONIC PANCREATITIS is an inflammation of the pancreas, an organ that secretes digestive enzymes and insulin. Pancreatitis is usually caused by heavy alcohol use or gallstones. Symptoms include severe abdominal and back pain, nausea, and fever. People with this condition are at risk for infection.

OSTEOARTHRITIS is the chronic presence of inflammation in a joint, usually as the result of damaged tissue. The cartilage designed to protect the bones from rubbing against each other often begins to erode with normal wear and tear, or as the result of an injury.

CHRONIC BRONCHITIS refers to an inflammation of the bronchial tubes, which join the windpipe to the lungs. Acute bronchitis, which lasts for about ten days, usually follows a virus or a cold, and will go away with proper treatment. The chronic form of this disease may be caused by repeated exposure to an irritant, like cigarette smoke, chemicals, dust, and allergens. Chronic bronchitis is one of the diseases that falls under the general category of chronic obstructive pulmonary disease, or COPD.

EMPHYSEMA, like chronic bronchitis, is categorized as a chronic obstructive pulmonary disease. It is a chronic inflammatory lung disease caused by smoking, or by air, environmental, or chemical pollutants. In this case, inflammation attacks the alveoli deep in the lungs, reducing the ability of the lungs to oxygenate the blood. In people with emphysema, the lung tissues necessary to support the physical shape and function of the lung are eventually destroyed by inflammation.

The Obesity Connection—Again?

The two diseases we've showcased as emblematic of the second category of diseases, heart disease and diabetes, are also ones that we strongly associate with obesity. That's not accidental. In fact, these two diseases again give us an opportunity to examine more closely the connection between inflammation and obesity—and how these two factors collide, in the case of these two diseases.

Let's look first at diabetes. Obesity and insulin resistance go hand in hand. Overweight people have high levels of fatty acids in their blood, and

Inflammatory Messenger Production
in Tissues of Healthy and Obese People

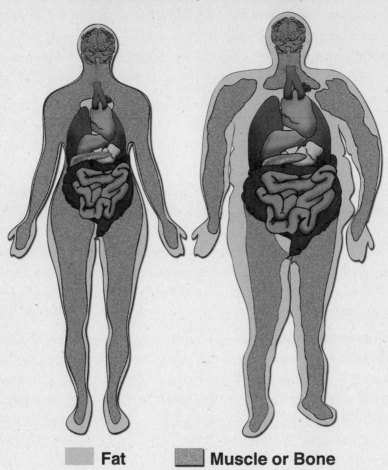

███ **Fat**   ███ **Muscle or Bone**

Comparison of Inflammatory Messengers
in Various Organ Tissues

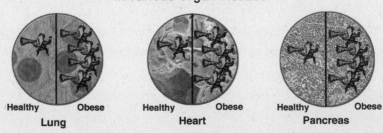

Healthy   Obese   Healthy   Obese   Healthy   Obese
Lung   **Heart**   **Pancreas**

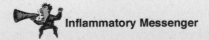 **Inflammatory Messenger**

a high level of fatty acids is one of the factors known to cause insulin resistance. In fact, most of the animal studies in this area use omega-6 fatty acids—the same fatty acids we know we eat too much of in the standard American diet—to trigger insulin resistance. It's no surprise, given what we eat, that insulin resistance is such a growing concern in this country.

In addition, the fatter we are, the more inflammatory messengers our fat cells make, and those inflammatory messengers cause insulin resistance, which leads to diabetes. *That's* how diabetes ends up being an inflammatory disease.

There's also a strong correlation between carrying excess weight and heart disease. This fits in with our understanding of heart disease as a lipid-storage problem: the same things you were eating that were making you fat were clogging your arteries. But here, too, the overlap between overweight and inflammation may also play a part. The fatter you are, the more inflammatory messengers you're making, which has the potential to worsen atherosclerosis. But that's not the only link.

Remember adiponectin, from chapter 2? It's a hormone with powerful anti-inflammatory properties, and people who are overweight produce considerably less of it. Adiponectin also prevents the transformation of white blood cells into foam cells, which play a critical role in the narrowing of the arteries, a leading factor in heart disease and heart attack. This may explain why having low levels of adiponectin in the blood—as many overweight people do—is associated with increased rates of heart disease.

Diseases in Which Overactive Inflammation Is *Suspected*

Now that inflammation is clearly emerging as a factor (if not the principal driving force) in such a wide range of human diseases, researchers are looking for it more and more—and they're finding it, often in very surprising places, such as the diseases in this third category.

Alzheimer's Dementia

This is a progressive neurodegenerative disease that is responsible for most cases of dementia in affluent countries. Symptoms of **Alzheimer's** include memory loss, an inability to speak, confusion, disorientation, restlessness, and mood swings.

There has been a pronounced rise in the disease over the past few decades, and the number of Americans with the disease is expected to triple by the year 2050.

Over the past few years, scientific investigators have begun to realize that some of the events associated with Alzheimer's disease are indicative of inflammation. It took longer than it might have to put the pieces of the puzzle together because the brain is protected by what's called the "blood-brain barrier," a kind of moat that protects the brain from substances in the blood. It was surprising to discover that inflammation could cross that blood-brain barrier.

However, the brain does have its own inflammatory-like cells, which are very similar to a type of white blood cell. Remarkably, these brain cells produce practically the same inflammatory messengers as the white blood cells.

Right now, there is not yet a large enough body of data for the scientific community to say definitively that Alzheimer's disease is, strictly speaking, an inflammatory disease. There are unquestionably inflammatory components. A current theory posits that the inflammatory process that drives Alzheimer's is very similar to the process that causes atherosclerosis. It has been suggested that the destruction of small blood vessels in the brain causes Alzheimer's, in very much the same way that the inflammatory process described above destroys blood vessels in the heart to cause heart disease.

The connection is further strengthened by the following observation: people who have taken anti-inflammatory drugs for a long period of time to treat another condition, like arthritis, have a reduced risk of contracting Alzheimer's.

Cancer

You probably don't think about cancer and inflammation together. In fact, many scientists don't either—yet. On their surfaces, the underlying mechanisms leading to inflammatory diseases and to cancer seem different, and yet clear links between these two conditions are emerging every day. This is at the very edge of research, and more must be done to determine exactly how large a role inflammation plays in this disease. One thing is true: if addressing inflammation is proven to prevent or treat certain types of cancers, this will open vast new therapeutic avenues.

An editorial in the March 2001 issue of the *Journal of Experimental Medicine* said, "Chronic inflammation predisposes humans to carcinoma [cancer] in the breast, liver, large bowel, urinary bladder, prostate, gastric mucosa, ovary, and skin. A large body of data indicates that use of anti-inflammatory drugs [aspirin and other nonsteroidal drugs] reduces colon cancer risk by 40 to 50 percent, and that it may be preventative for lung, esophagus, and stomach cancer."

Cervical cancer is another cancer that may have an inflammatory component. It is often the result of human papillomavirus (HPV) or other sexually transmitted diseases like herpes, gonorrhea, or chlamydia. These STDs cause an inflammation of the cervix, which may contribute to the cell changes that result in cancer.

It's difficult to be more specific about the exact role that inflammation plays in this third category of diseases; the science just isn't there yet. As a result, it's hard to know whether the Chilton Program might play an effective role in their treatment. We are right on the cutting edge of this research, and I have every expectation that we will soon have a much fuller picture of how anti-inflammatory strategies, including medications and the Chilton Program, can help those at risk and those who suffer from these diseases.

Even People with Inflammatory Disease Are at Further Risk!

Treating your disease by addressing the underlying inflammation serves more than one purpose. First of all, it will lessen the symptoms and severity of your disease—a hugely important factor. But it will also protect you against developing other inflammatory diseases by curbing your body's destructive hypersensitivity. Let me explain. When the volume control on your immune system is turned up too high, the reverberations are felt throughout your body, not just in the area where your inflammatory disease is concentrated.

This is why so many of these diseases seem to go hand in hand: people with psoriasis, for instance, often suffer from asthma and arthritis. If the overall level of inflammation in the body is too high, every system is at risk. Thus overactive inflammation must be cut off at the pass.

> Having one inflammatory condition puts you at much greater risk of contracting another.

We must treat the *cause* of these diseases instead of simply addressing their symptoms. Taking a medication to treat the symptoms of one inflammatory disease does nothing to suppress the overall level of inflammation in your body. As a result, you're vulnerable to attack from another quarter.

Is There More to Come?

Asthma. Psoriasis. Heart disease. Lupus. Eczema. Psoriasis. Diabetes. Inflammatory bowel disease. Arthritis. It's an incredible variety of diseases that can be clustered under the single umbrella of inflammation.

Now I must send up a further alarm: I personally believe that this seemingly random "laundry list" of inflammatory diseases is about to get much longer.

A few years ago, during a game of hospital, my young daughter, Sarah, diagnosed her beloved teddy bear, Little Lucy, with a bad case of "bearitis." I've heard that old nursery chestnut a thousand times (I have four children), but for the first time, I really *heard* it. *Itis,* in case you don't know, comes from the Greek word for inflammation. My daughter's automatic use of "itis" as a suffix to diagnose her teddy bear made me realize just how synonymous—how closely joined, and inextricably linked—inflammation is with disease.

> The diseases we now categorize as inflammatory may be only the tip of the iceberg.

As research progresses, we are discovering how right my daughter was. Inflammation is, in fact, inextricably linked to disease, and the diseases that we categorize as inflammatory disease may be just the tip of the iceberg.

Many of the diseases in the second and third categories are an indication that change is afoot. In fact, the categories above are more of a reflection of the "state of the science"—what researchers know about the role inflammation plays in these diseases—than about the pathology of the diseases themselves.

In other words, just because a disease falls in the second or third category doesn't mean that inflammation is any less of an important factor in causing it than it is for a disease in the first category. It simply means that this is where scientists feel comfortable categorizing it, given the medical community's current state of knowledge.

In another five years, at the pace new knowledge is being acquired, it is very possible that a disease could move from the second category, a disease where inflammation is known to be a primary component, to the first, a disease *caused* by inflammation.

I call this the inflammatory continuum.

You can see how fluid these categories are simply by referring back to the heart disease and Alzheimer's disease examples discussed earlier. No one thought these diseases had anything to do with inflammation: now we know it plays an important part. More often than not, as research emerges, inflammation is shown to have a more prominent role than originally believed.

From a scientific perspective, it's a fascinating time to be in this field. But it's also frightening. As the number of diseases in these categories increases, so does the number of people affected by them. And if you believe, as I do, that something in our environment is contributing to this inflammatory epidemic, then every single one of us is unwittingly threatening our, and our family's, health.

The Silver Lining

As harrowing as it might seem that all these diseases, no matter how different from one another they might seem, share the same underlying menace, there is a silver lining to the commonality as well. If the Chilton Program has cracked the code that controls overactive inflammation, then we stand a very good chance of preventing, treating, and even reversing *many* of these diseases.

> If we unlock the secret to controlling overactive inflammation, we can prevent, treat, and even reverse many of these diseases.

In the next chapter, you'll see how the Chilton Program stops inflammation, using the same gold-standard science that has given way to the most powerful wave of anti-inflammatory medications in the history of medicine.

Chapter Four
The Billion-Dollar Pathway

Imagine a broad spectrum, over-the-counter product that relieves pain caused by everything from headaches to muscle strain and reduces dangerously high fevers. Now imagine that this simple pill has also emerged as an important force in preventing the blood clots that cause stroke and heart attack, and that it has, researchers believe, an important preventative role in colon, breast, and other cancers as well.

You don't have to imagine such a drug—it already exists. It's aspirin, and it's probably in your medicine cabinet right now.

Aspirin is amazing, and not just because of its versatility and efficacy. The scientific exploration of the secrets behind this wonder drug led to one of the single most important discoveries of the twentieth century from an inflammatory perspective: the discovery of the AA Pathway.

The Medium Is the Message

We know from chapter 2 that the inflammatory messengers called leukotrienes and prostaglandins control major aspects of the immune system's inflammatory response.

These inflammatory messengers control the *intensity* of the attack by requesting that white blood cells come to the site of infection or injury. They control the *collateral damage* done during that attack, by concentrating the white blood cell army in certain areas of the tissue, and they control *how long the attack lasts,* by helping the white blood cells to stay alive longer than they would on their own.

Too many of these messengers, and our immune system overreacts with devastating consequences.

Blocking the Billion-Dollar Pathway

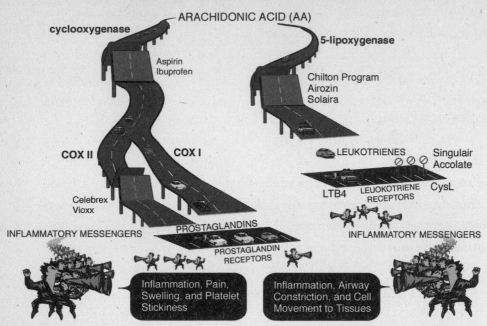

Here, then, is the crux of the problem. The reason we're facing an unprecedented epidemic of inflammatory disease in this country—and in all first-world countries—is that, for some reason, extraordinarily large numbers of us are producing an overabundance of these and other inflammatory messengers.

> When we produce too many inflammatory messengers, our inflammatory response becomes too severe, and too protracted—which results in chronic inflammatory disease.

The question that remains to be answered if we are going to reverse this terrible trend—and prevent it in those who have been lucky enough thus far to dodge the bullet—is whether or not we can do something to prevent this exaggerated response. Can we block the production of these inflammatory messengers so that we're making enough to defend ourselves against disease and infection, yet not making too many?

The search for the answer to this very question has spawned a massive investment on the part of the pharmaceutical industry, which has spent billions of dollars in search of a "magic bullet," one that can control the overproduction of these inflammatory messengers. Although we don't yet have that magic bullet, the investment has already paid off richly, both for the companies funding the research and for their beneficiaries, sufferers of inflammatory disease.

First of all, their research has led to the most powerful wave of anti-inflammatory medications humankind has ever seen, drugs that have now become household names, like Celebrex and Singulair. These drugs have saved many lives, and they have improved the quality of many more.

As you will see in this chapter, that same research also opened the door to a whole new approach to treating inflammation—the Chilton Program, a natural approach that is nevertheless grounded in hard science, and that operates along the very same pathway as those blockbuster drugs. As you'll see, this natural, scientifically based dietary program does what these drugs do, and more.

Take Two and Call Me in the Morning

The discovery of the AA Pathway began as a medical mystery thousands of years old.

Salicylic acid is a substance derived from the bark of the willow tree, and it is the reason that willow bark has been a successful component in various "remedies" for thousands of years. Used by the Egyptians and the Sumerians to treat the symptoms of rheumatism, willow bark was mentioned by Hippocrates, "the father of medicine," in 400 B.C. for use as a painkiller during childbirth. In 1763, the Reverend Edmund Stone, a British vicar, gave the first description of its effects in a letter, and scientists across Europe worked to create an analgesic from this bark.

More than a hundred years later, a German chemist named Felix Hoffman managed to synthesize a drug that had all of the painkilling and anti-inflammatory aspects of salicylic acid, with a buffer to reduce the stomach irritation it caused. We know that drug, made while Hoffman was in the employ of a company called Bayer, as aspirin.

The new drug skyrocketed to become the most widely relied-upon medication in history, because it worked so well and on such a wide range of problems. Still, in spite of its wide usage, no one knew precisely how it worked—and wouldn't, until almost a century later.

In 1971, Sir John Vane, a British researcher, and his colleagues discovered that aspirin and similar drugs produced their effects because they inhibited the production of certain inflammatory messengers called prostaglandins. These inflammatory messengers play a central role in the inflammation story: they encourage the blood vessels to dilate, resulting in the swelling and redness of inflammation, and they stimulate the nerve endings that send pain messages to the brain.

The Villain of the Inflammatory Story

How do these inflammatory messengers come into being? These messengers—prostaglandins and leukotrienes—are synthesized from an omega-6 fatty acid called arachidonic acid, or AA. Obviously, some level of AA is necessary so that the body's immune system is not left defenseless. But when we have too much AA, we produce too many inflammatory messengers; too many messengers, and we have inflammatory disease.

The production of inflammatory messengers from this fatty acid is called the AA Pathway, and this single pathway is the starting point for a critical component of inflammation—whether that inflammation is an appropriate response to danger, or the result of an inflammatory system on overdrive, as it is in inflammatory disease.

Vane's discovery of how aspirin worked was revolutionary. We had known that prostaglandins were a product of the AA Pathway, but his research showed us the mechanism by which the production of inflammatory messengers through this pathway could be *blocked*.

Let me explain. In order for AA to turn into prostaglandins, it has to go through a chemical process, which I like to compare to cooking. Throw tomatoes, onions, garlic, and some oregano into a pot to simmer, and in a little while you'll have your grandmother's marinara sauce. But without the heat of the stove, the individual elements can't, and won't, blend together to make the sauce.

Vane demonstrated that aspirin (and drugs like it) block a crucial enzyme, or a chemical key, called cyclooxygenase, or COX. This enzyme helps AA turn into prostaglandins. Aspirin, in a sense, blows out the pilot light, and if AA can't get together with the enzyme it needs, it can't turn into prostaglandins.

In other words, aspirin cuts pain and inflammation off at the pass by preventing those inflammatory messengers from being produced. This is why it's such a "wonder drug," useful for everything from relieving muscle stiffness and headaches, to preventing heart disease. Vane and his colleagues won a Nobel Prize in Medicine in 1982 for their work. The impact of their research simply cannot be overestimated, and it continues to be felt today.

The AA Pathway Strikes Again

Meanwhile, another team led by two investigators, Sune Bergstrom and Bengt Samuelsson, was working on another line of research that would push our understanding of the mechanism behind inflammation even further. These scientists had identified a substance in the lungs of asthmatics which they called "the slow-reacting substance of anaphylaxis." When this substance was removed and put into the lungs of dogs, it was shown to cause the same signs and symptoms of asthma—inflammation, constriction and blockage of the airways, movement of white blood cells into the lungs—in the animals as it did in humans.

Figuring out exactly what this substance was, how it was made, and how it worked, took almost a decade, and part of the 1982 Nobel Prize in Medicine was also awarded to these scientists for their work. It turned out that this slow-reacting substance of anaphylaxis was made up of another family of inflammatory messengers, called leukotrienes. These leukotrienes were a thousand times more potent than histamine, the central messenger that had already been isolated in asthmatics.

And leukotrienes, a key driving force behind many inflammatory diseases including asthma, Crohn's disease, heart disease, and arthritis, were different from prostaglandins, but they were produced from the same fatty acid pathway: the AA Pathway.

Together, these discoveries—how these inflammatory messengers were made from AA, and how this AA Pathway could be interrupted—were landmarks. They meant that we could work toward blocking inflammatory messengers, which brought us one step closer to being able to help people who suffer from devastating inflammatory diseases.

Anti-Inflammatory Medications: A Road Paved with Gold

Scientists in pharmaceutical companies, as well as in medical centers funded by government organizations such as the National Institutes of Health, have spent billions of dollars on research to develop medications that short-circuit this AA Pathway. The fruits of their labors fall into two categories: the drugs that block prostaglandins, and the drugs that block leukotrienes.

The Prostaglandin Blockers

Some of these medications draw directly on Sir John Vane's research, bringing pain relief by blocking prostaglandins.

You might be wondering, Why do we need new prostaglandin blockers when we know that's what aspirin does?

Unfortunately, aspirin, for all its effectiveness (and despite Felix Hoffman's buffer), isn't side-effect free. In the 1990s, two scientific teams (in one of which I was a part) discovered that there are two types of COX enzymes, the enzymes that turn AA into prostaglandins. The first, COX-1, is responsible for a number of maintenance and housekeeping functions in the body. One of these housekeeping chores is maintaining the thickness of the stomach lining. The other, COX-2, is the one behind much of the pain and inflammation.

Aspirin isn't specific: it blocks both COX enzymes, which means that it prevents COX-1 from doing its housekeeping job, even as it stops pain and inflammation. So when you take aspirin, your stomach lining suffers—sometimes to the point of serious pain and bleeding, symptoms that grow progressively worse over time.

Obviously, this isn't a workable situation, so the drug companies worked hard to develop more selective medications that would block only COX-2, leaving the stomach lining more intact. You know these COX-2 inhibitors as drugs like Vioxx and Celebrex. However, these medications are not entirely free of side effects. In fact, a very recent study was published indicating that patients taking the COX-2 inhibitor Vioxx had, after eighteen months, an increased risk for confirmed cardiovascular events such as heart attack and stroke, when compared to those taking a placebo. Vioxx has now been removed from the marketplace; more studies will be necessary to determine whether this serious side effect is specific to Vioxx or extends to other COX-2 inhibitors.

The Leukotriene Blockers

Another category of anti-inflammatory medication that came about as a result of the research into the AA Pathway was the leukotriene blockers, so called because they prevent leukotrienes, our other type of inflammatory messenger from AA, from signalling inflammatory cells.

These medications, like Singulair and Accolate, have also gained astonishing popularity since their development. Singulair alone had sales exceeding $2 billion in 2003, an increase of 35 percent from 2002. Unfortunately, although they are wonderful medications and have brought an enormous amount of relief to many people, these drugs can block only one type of leukotriene, not the whole family of leukotrienes. If you've had less than completely satisfactory results on these medications, it's probably because they weren't blocking the type of leukotriene that causes your disease.

How the Chilton Program Complements Your Treatment Path

While pharmaceutical companies were backing scientists with hundreds of millions of dollars to discover the industry's next wave of blockbuster drugs, I was determined to use my funding from the National Institutes of Health to explore whether a dietary solution might do the same job. Not only was the science compelling, but I had seen up close—and recent studies confirm—the toll taken on the body when chronic sufferers become dependent on powerful drugs for relief.

I certainly do not oppose the use of medications, especially in treatment for inflammatory disease. These medications are literally lifesavers for millions of people, my sister and my son among them. I don't think anyone with real experience with these diseases can make an argument against drugs that relieve as much pain and restore as much quality of life for sufferers as these do. Indeed, I worked on many of the studies that gave rise to some of these blockbuster drugs, and I applaud the pharmaceutical industry for their continued research in this area.

That aside, I don't think I'm shocking anyone by saying that these medications are far from perfect: there is still no pharmaceutical solution for inflammatory disease. Surely anything that can give these medications a boost will be a welcome addition to the field.

I encourage you—truly—to think of the Chilton Program as a *complementary* strategy, not an alternative one. You don't need to choose. The Chilton Program is designed to assist and improve the results from your medication. It is always a physician's goal to reduce dosages, or to wean a patient off medication entirely—but only if that is a realistic goal. With lifesaving medications like the ones available, no one should be in pain, or should suffer advancement of his or her disease because of the pursuit of a natural solution.

A Side-Effect-Free Solution

One of the most compelling arguments for finding a dietary solution to this epidemic of epidemics is the need for relief without side effects.

Every drug has some side effects. Whenever your doctor prescribes a medication, he or she weighs the potential benefits of that medication against the discomfort or damage that the side effects are likely to cause. This is called a risk-benefit ratio, and it is a factor doctors take into account every single time they pull out a prescription pad.

This is why cancer patients are often prescribed medications that would be considered poisons if they were administered to a healthy person. These drugs come with severe side effects, but their lifesaving potential outweighs the risks.

This risk-benefit ratio is an issue whenever a medication is prescribed, but it is a special issue when we're talking about chronic diseases (like many of the inflammatory diseases). In many of these cases, if you have a chronic inflammatory disease, and you've been prescribed a medication, you're going on it for a prolonged period of time—maybe even for life. So your physician always has to be mindful of the long-term side effects of your medications.

Worse, many of these diseases are progressive, forcing patients and their physicians into an ever-escalating series of ever-worsening medication choices. One of the things that strikes me whenever I'm in a room with a group of inflammatory disease sufferers is how much of their conversation deals not with their diseases, but with managing the side effects of their medications.

Take Jennifer, who was diagnosed with a mild-to-moderate case of rheumatoid arthritis. Her doctor put her on Celebrex, a COX-2 non-steroidal anti-inflammatory drug (NSAID), to manage her morning stiffness and some of the discomfort she was feeling in her knees and elbows. COX-2 NSAIDs are better for the stomach than the COX-1 family, for sure, but they're not entirely side-effect free. Again, very recent studies suggest there may be more side effects than originally thought. In any event, Jennifer's doctor wasn't surprised when she began to experience stomach upset after about a year of taking her medicine.

Jennifer managed her RA (and the gastrointestinal side effects of her NSAID) for another year with some discomfort, when a sudden, painful flare-up in her disease stopped her in her tracks just before her son's wedding.

In response, her doctor recommended treatment with steroids to stabilize her condition. These steroids are not the same steroids that athletes abuse to increase their performance level—those are *anabolic* steroids. These *cortico*steroids, like prednisolone, are used in the treatment of all forms of moderate-to-severe inflammatory disease. They are very effective at stopping inflammation, although they take their toll in side effects over the short term, and *especially* over the long. I once remarked to a colleague that we could probably alleviate most symptoms of inflammatory disease if we could give high enough doses of steroids for long enough periods of time. He wryly responded that the patient would certainly experience relief—either because the steroids had successfully stopped the inflammation, or because their side effects had killed him.

Jennifer's doctor tried to keep her on the lowest steroid dose possible, but her short-term side effects were practically textbook nonetheless. She experienced weight gain, an upset stomach, easy bruising, and mood shifts, including a fairly serious depression. After doing a little research on long-term side effects, which can include osteoporosis, diabetes, and the permanent suppression of the adrenal gland, she felt greatly relieved that she'd be on the medication only until the flare passed.

The long-term effects of high doses of steroids aren't good. Here's why: steroids aren't selective. When you take a steroid, the drug infiltrates the nucleus of *every single one* of your cells, and starts monkeying around with the genes it finds there. It probably plays with hundreds of genes.

A small number of these genes controls the pain and inflammation associated with inflammatory diseases; steroids turn many of these genes off, which is a good thing. However, because steroids are not selective, they also regulate the genes that control kidney, liver, brain, and heart function—which is *not* a good thing. It is likely that steroid treatment plays with other genes, too, including genes we don't know a lot about right now. So in a sense, we're waiting for the other shoe to drop.

In diseases like asthma, we can reduce many of the risks of steroid use by using an inhaler, which means the steroid is localized in the lungs. In other inflammatory diseases, like Jennifer's arthritis (and even in asthma when the disease becomes severe), you have to take the drug internally, so it pervades the entire body, which increases the likelihood of short-term side effects and long-term damage.

Unfortunately, Jennifer's repeated attempts to stop using the steroid were unsuccessful. Her disease worsened to the point at which she wasn't able to be off the drug for any amount of time without experiencing painful flare-ups. Over the next two years, her disease continued its downward spiral until, finally, even the steroids were no longer fully controlling it. Many days now, her pain is so severe that it's not possible for her to function normally at all.

Jennifer is now exploring with her doctor other options like methotrexate, a cancer drug that can be effective in slowing the progress of the disease, but can also do very serious damage to the kidneys and liver. Together, they're considering Enbrel, also very effective, although it's been linked to several long-term side effects, including serious infections.

Here you can see the risk-benefit ratio in action. As Jennifer's disease and symptoms worsen, the medications she must take to alleviate her symptoms and halt her disease become more serious, with ever more severe side effects.

I believe the Chilton Program can help, by providing Jennifer and her doctor with a supplemental treatment plan that has the potential to make a very big difference in her long-term health.

And I'm sure Jennifer will notice a tremendous difference in the way she feels, once she starts eating delicious and healthy foods, perfectly calibrated for her body's needs. I'm willing to bet that the difference won't just be in her inflammatory disease symptoms, but in her overall health and outlook.

Don't be fooled. A remedy doesn't have to cause noxious side effects to present a powerful solution. We've gotten so accustomed to the toll that effective medications take on us that we're mistrustful of anything that doesn't exact such a toll. But, as you'll see, the truth in this instance is that this safe and all-natural approach may even work *more* effectively than heavy-duty medications with their heavy-duty side effects.

> A remedy doesn't have to cause noxious side effects to present a powerful solution.

A Full-Spectrum Blocker

Here's why: when you meet the needs of your body by giving it the food it needs in the right balance, you can do naturally what no medication has been able to do, despite the billions spent on research.

Let's look at the leukotriene blockers, for instance. Some of the most popular medications on the market, like Singulair, are effective against only one specific leukotriene. This is great news if that leukotriene is the one causing your inflammatory condition, and not such good news if a different one is the underlying culprit.

By contrast, the Chilton Program is able to inhibit the production of the *entire family* of leukotrienes. Doctors—and pharmaceutical companies—have been saying for years that they'd love to get their hands on a magic bullet, something that works as a general inhibitor for the full class of leukotrienes. This is precisely what my diet was designed to do. By controlling the balance of the fatty acids we consume, it delivers a full-sweep block of these inflammatory messengers.

> The Chilton Program does what no drug on the market can do, by offering a full-spectrum block of the AA Pathway.

In one of several pivotal clinical trials we did at Wake Forest University School of Medicine, we showed that by applying the rules of the Chilton Program to asthmatics, we could inhibit leukotriene production in the vast majority of asthma patients. For example, the results of this study showed that we succeeded in suppressing the production of leukotrienes in 78 percent of the asthma sufferers. In other words, we saw a 78 percent success rate. This result far exceeded even our own expectations.

And not only did our program block *all* (not some!) leukotrienes, but it did so more effectively in the 50 percent of asthmatics who produced the highest level of leukotrienes. In other words, it most helped the people who needed it most—often the people whose medications leave them out in the cold.

Treating the Disease, Not Just the Symptoms

Although I am not, for a minute, minimizing their benefits, it is clear that medications are not a complete solution for inflammatory disease sufferers.

Is there any solution apart from these medications to combat inflammatory messengers? While drugs such as Singular and Accolate perform a very important role, they don't address the root cause of these diseases, the *production* of inflammatory messengers.

Even when a leukotriene blocker works for you, it's not really stopping the body's inappropriate response to harmless intruders like pollen and pet dander. Instead, you experience relief because the degree of that inappropriate response is reduced. That's an improvement, but it's not a solution. You don't want your toddler to have *less* of a ferocious tantrum when his peas touch his carrots, you want him not to have the tantrum at all.

We must now do more than treat the symptoms; this pandemic cannot be solved with Band-Aids. We must address the underlying condition that is causing our own bodies to rise up against us in this destructive manner.

Because the simple truth is that inflammatory diseases can be—and often are—fatal. I'm not overstating the case. The life expectancy of a rheumatoid arthritis sufferer is shorter than someone's in the general population. People die from scleroderma. They die from asthma. And they are dying in record numbers right now, numbers that continue to climb, despite the improvements in medical technology, including these medications.

Stopping Inflammation Before It Starts

I'm grateful that this new wave of anti-inflammatory medications is there for those who have inflammatory disease, but I believe that we need to address the underlying *cause* of overactive inflammation. We can do that, not simply by interrupting the AA Pathway, as medications do, but by stopping it before it starts.

We can set a broken leg, but isn't prevention of the injury really the wiser course? We began this chapter wondering whether it was possible to block inflammatory messengers, and as we've seen, it is, at least some of the time. But isn't a better question whether it's possible to intervene even earlier, so that we don't see an overproduction of inflammatory messengers in the first place—and therefore have no need to block them? Is there a course correction we can make in our lifestyles, both individually and in the country as a whole, that can help us to normalize our production of these messengers?

Can we stop the AA Pathway before it starts?

It gives me tremendous pleasure to say, after years of research, that I believe the answer to the question is a resounding *yes*. Now that we understand many of the intricate mechanisms by which our diet regulates the AA Pathway, we can begin to bring our overproduction of these in-flammatory messengers under control. And that yes has wide-reaching and important ramifications in all of our lives. Although we are all at risk, we need not all fall victim.

I also believe that yes means we can bring needed relief to people who suffer from horrendously painful and debilitating inflammatory diseases. And, finally, that yes means that we can begin to pull our Inflammation Nation out of its nosedive by protecting ourselves and our families from the looming threat of these diseases.

The Chilton Program—my all-natural, easy-to-follow, dietary approach—combats out-of-control inflammation in two ways:

Like the blockbuster prescription drugs Singulair and Accolate, the first principle of the Chilton Program is to block inflammatory messengers, like leukotrienes, from signaling inflammatory cells.

The Chilton Program has a distinct advantage over those medications, because it gives your body the weapons it needs to block *many different types* of leukotrienes, each one carrying its own inflammatory message. In contrast, Singulair and Accolate block only one type of leukotriene, and that specific leukotriene's message, from interacting with your body's inflammatory cells. So this dietary solution blocks a wider array of inflammatory messengers, which control a broad range of disease signs and symptoms.

But the power of the Chilton Program doesn't stop there. It inhibits inflammation *before it starts* by reducing the number of building blocks that give rise to inflammatory messengers.

By reducing the material with which inflammatory messengers are made, the Chilton Program *prevents* overactive inflammation. This second key principle presents, for the first time, a preemptive solution to inflammatory disease. Inflammatory disease comes about because your body produces too many inflammatory messengers, with the result that your inflammatory system is set on a hair trigger: all too ready to launch a full-scale attack against something innocuous, like an allergen or your body's own tissue. Your body needs certain building blocks to make these

> The Chilton Program inhibits inflammation *before it starts.*

messengers. By reducing the number of those building blocks, we reduce the number of inappropriate signals the body can send. So instead of waiting until the cells are cocked and fully loaded, ready for the trigger to be pulled, the Chilton Program starts even further back in the process. By taking some of those building blocks out of our blood, we're effectively removing some of the bullets from the gun.

What We've Learned, So Far

How can simple dietary changes have such tremendous effects—effects greater, in some cases, than the results you can get with some of the very best and most sophisticated medications on the market?

Let's take a moment to review what we know. We know that an overabundance of inflammatory messengers plays a major role in causing inflammatory disease. We know that our body produces these inflammatory messengers from a fatty acid called AA (arachidonic acid). We know that high levels of this fatty acid cause the overproduction of inflammatory messengers.

Too much AA causes us to produce too many inflammatory messengers, and too many inflammatory messengers cause the signs and symptoms of inflammatory disease.

Doesn't it then make sense that controlling the levels of AA in the blood is one key to controlling overactive inflammation?

To understand this clearly we must dig a little more deeply into the very genesis of the inflammatory process to answer the next logical question:

How can we reduce the amount of AA in our bodies? Where are the high levels of this fatty acid coming from? Stick with me here: I can assure you that I'll make it worth your while.

The Skinny on Fat

In order to find the source of these high levels of AA, we'll need to take a closer look at what you know—and what you *think* you know—about fats. This is by no means a rehash of the "good fat/bad fat" debate so familiar to health-conscious consumers. Indeed, our discovery will force us to take a whole new look at this macronutrient.

The American public has been at the receiving end of a tremendous and ongoing campaign of misinformation about fats. In the 1980s, all fats were considered "bad." Wave after wave of low-fat or fat-free (and sugar-heavy!) products hit the grocery shelves. In the 1990s, the general public learned to differentiate between saturated fat, the kind found in animal products, and the more heart-healthy unsaturated fats, like those found in olive oil, avocados, and almonds. Saturated fats were perceived as "bad," unsaturated fats as "good."

More recently, we've been able to add another level of sophistication to our knowledge. We now know that not all unsaturated fats are created equal. The polyunsaturated fats (PUFAs) can be divided into two categories: the omega-3 fatty acids (such as the ones found in fatty fish), and the omega-6 fatty acids (such as the ones found in soybean oil). Several diets out there, including some designed by the most famous doctors, will tell you that all omega-3s are the "good" fats, and all omega-6s are the "bad" ones. Although it is true that we eat too many of certain omega-6 fatty acids, and not enough of certain omega-3s, my own scientific research directly challenges the wisdom of dividing these fats into strictly positive and negative categories.

The omega-3 and omega-6 fatty acids are called "essential fatty acids" because we need to get them from food. Our body can't make them—and without them, we risk heart, brain, and liver disorders; growth retardation; sterility; a susceptibility to infections; and the impairment of our vision as well as emotional and learning disabilities.

Although we can't make these fatty acids, we can convert them into other fatty acids once we've eaten them. This conversion process is like playing with Lego or Duplo blocks. We change fatty acids by putting them through a chemical process involving enzymes that adds bends or additional length to their structure.

Let's take a look at how this process works by focusing for a moment on one specific fat. Linoleic acid (LA) is, by far, the most plentiful omega-6 fatty acid in our diets. It's in almost everything we eat that contains fat, including meat, most seed oils, dairy products, and eggs. When there's a lot of this fatty acid in the body (as there always is in Western diets), we change this fatty acid into another omega-6 fatty acid called gammalinolenic acid, or GLA. We do this by putting another bend in the fatty-acid unit.

Now, our bodies limit the process, so only a small amount of LA gets changed into GLA.

We can then change GLA, by lengthening the fatty acid unit a little, into another fatty acid called DGLA, which stands for dihomogamma-linolenic acid. We're a little better at this conversion, so it goes a little faster. Another bend in the fatty acid unit and DGLA is converted to AA, the arachidonic acid we discussed earlier. So this alphabet soup of fatty-acid conversions—from LA to GLA to DGLA to AA—is one way in which we end up with AA in our bloodstream.

Does this mean that if you want to stop making so much AA, you should stop eating LA? Actually, it doesn't. A number of recent studies indicate that we convert very little LA into AA. Our bodies aren't good at the first conversion of LA to GLA. Consequently, eating even a lot of LA (as almost all of us do every day) won't really have a major influence on AA, or on the number of inflammatory messengers you produce.

We didn't always know this—for a very simple reason. Not all species so limit this conversion. Rodents, including mice, are actually very good at it, which means that they convert a great deal of the LA they eat into AA. So what? Many of the studies examining how the body processes different fatty acids were carried out in mice, which means that some of the conclusions scientists drew about the connection between dietary LA and elevated levels of AA *in humans* were incorrect. These experiments did answer some important questions, but these mice also added a great deal of confusion to the scientific understanding of how humans process these fatty acids.

The Trickle-Down Theory

Let's move back to humans—and our ongoing mystery: how does AA get into our bloodstreams at such terribly elevated levels? LA would have made a convenient villain, since it's so prevalent in our diet, but our own inefficiency at making those fatty-acid conversions lessens its importance. We have to look somewhere else for our answer.

I like to use an analogy to explain the way our bodies move through this series of fatty-acid conversions. Think about a series of buckets, one on top of another, each with a hole in the bottom, dripping liquid into the bucket below it. The topmost bucket, of course, is LA. When we eat a lot of this omega-6, it's as if we're pouring a lot of liquid into that bucket. In industrialized countries, that's pretty much all the time, so imagine that we start by eating a big meal, which fills that top bucket, marked LA, to the brim.

Now we know that the human body converts a small amount of LA into GLA, right? So GLA is our second bucket, which sits below the LA bucket. At the bottom of the LA bucket is a small hole, which allows a small quantity of liquid into the GLA bucket right below it. Below the GLA bucket is our DGLA bucket—and because our bodies are a little better at converting GLA into DGLA, the hole at the bottom of that bucket is a little bigger, so there's a slightly faster dribble of liquid into the

Dietary AA and Inflammatory Messengers

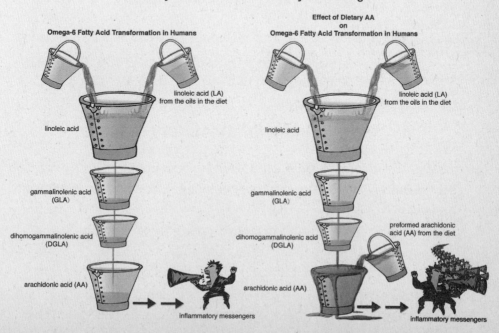

DGLA bucket. Beneath the DGLA bucket is the AA bucket. Here the amount slows again, because our bodies tightly control putting the next bend in the fatty acid. So the stream going from the DGLA bucket into that last AA bucket is little more than a trickle.

Because the holes are small, we're talking about a small amount of liquid in each of the subsequent buckets, especially by the time we get to that final bucket, the AA bucket at the bottom of the tier. A small amount of AA in the bottom bucket isn't a bad thing; it only results in normal levels of inflammatory messengers.

But, as we know, we don't just have a tiny bit of AA in our buckets. If we did, I don't believe we would be looking at inflammatory disease in such epidemic proportion. Instead, our AA buckets are filled to overflowing, with the result that we produce too many of the inflammatory messengers that lead to inflammatory disease.

Question: how does all that AA get into that bottom bucket?

Answer: *The same way all that LA got into the top one: we eat huge amounts of preformed AA in our Western diets.*

Every time we eat a meal filled with AA, we bypass all the other fatty-acid buckets and the conversions they represent, and we fill that bottom AA bucket directly, right up to the rim.

The food we eat is our most direct source of AA.

This is why our blood levels of AA are often high—and, I believe, one of the reasons we are facing an inflammatory epidemic at this time.

Dietary AA and Inflammatory Disease

There is a direct connection between the amount of preformed AA that we consume in our diets and the amount of inflammatory messengers that our body produces. Dr. Jay Whelan and his colleagues at the University of Tennessee and Cornell demonstrated in the early 1990s that introducing even low amounts of dietary AA into hamster diets caused a dramatic upsurge in the ability of inflammatory cells to produce inflammatory messengers.

The same is true in clinical trials done in humans. Dr. Andrew Sinclair and his colleagues in Australia have shown that the more dietary AA humans consume in foods, the more inflammatory messengers they produce. In fact, research has proven that a high AA diet has the potential actually to change normal immune responses to abnormal, exaggerated ones. A study carried out in 1997 by Dr. Darshan S. Kelley and colleagues at the Western Human Nutrition Research Center in California showed that people on high-AA diets generated *four times* as many inflammatory cells after a flu vaccination as people on low-AA diets.

> High levels of AA in our diets cause us to produce abnormally high numbers of inflammatory messengers.

Dietary AA and Heart Disease

Although researchers aren't completely sure how AA works to affect other body processes, there is a very strong connection between this inflammatory fatty acid and one of the most prevalent and serious inflammatory conditions: heart disease.

Platelet stickiness is an important risk factor for heart disease; it signals that someone with thickening of the arteries is at higher risk for a heart attack. In 1997, Dr. Aldo Ferretti and his colleagues at the Nutrition Requirements and Functions Laboratory did a study that showed that people on a high-AA diet (1,500 milligrams a day) had 41 percent more of the messengers that control inflammation *and* platelet stickiness than people on a low-AA diet, one that contained only 210 milligrams of AA per day.

Another, more recent study, published in the *New England Journal of Medicine* by Dr. Margaret Mehrabian's laboratory, further connected the dots between AA and heart disease. These scientists demonstrated that the enzyme that makes leukotrienes from AA in the human body is different than normal in some patients with atherosclerosis and related heart disease. Patients with this different enzyme have the much thicker artery walls associated with heart disease compared to patients without this different enzyme. This discovery indicates that there is a genetic predisposition to this disease that can be directly linked to the way AA is processed.

However, the most interesting finding in this study was that the atherosclerosis and related heart disease was made much worse in these patients if they ate diets that contained high levels of preformed AA. So lots of AA—whether because of its inflammatory potential or not—made heart disease much worse. This critical observation is backed up by three other studies in animals and humans.

What conclusions can we draw from these data? There is unquestionably a connection between elevated levels of AA in the diet and elevated levels in the blood. High levels of AA in the blood cause significant increases in a number of parameters that directly affect our health: the production, and overproduction, of inflammatory messengers, as well as the messengers that call for platelet aggregation, or stickiness, a major contributor to heart attack. In people cursed with a certain genetic makeup, eating high levels of AA dramatically leads to—and worsens—serious human diseases, like heart disease, the leading killer of Americans today.

These studies paint a very sobering picture of this omega-6 fatty acid, and I believe that there's a great deal more to come. I anticipate that we will soon know much more about the connection between a high level of AA in our diets and serious human inflammatory disease.

The Older We Get, the Worse It Gets

We already know that there is a strong connection between the AA in our diets and inflammatory conditions such as asthma and heart disease. But is AA the key to understanding why these diseases seem to manifest themselves so frequently in the elderly?

In chapter 1, I mentioned that one of the big theories I often hear to explain the inflammatory epidemic is that these are "diseases of old age." Improved medications and sanitary conditions have resulted in dramatically increased life spans.

Now I am convinced, mostly because children are the fastest-growing population affected by these diseases, that this "old age" theory is not actually the one that explains why we are currently experiencing this epidemic. But there may be some validity to the observation that these inflammatory diseases seem disproportionately to plague the elderly. In other words, people may not simply be getting these diseases because they're old—but it does seem as if a great number of old people are affected by them.

Don't we take the appearance of many of these diseases for granted as we age? It is true that a disease like osteoarthritis, caused in some part by wear and tear, is more likely to show up in someone who has logged sixty-plus years of that wear and tear on their joints. But perhaps here, too, AA plays a major role.

My laboratory has just published a paper in the *Journal of Nutritional Health and Aging* showing that the concentration of AA in our blood naturally increases as we age. To do the study, we took a group of younger and older adults, and we fed them ordinary Western diets. The food they ate was prepared in what's called a "metabolic kitchen," which means that all of the nutrients in each food item were carefully analyzed and portions strictly weighed before the participants ate the meals, to ensure that everyone was eating the same thing in the same amounts. When blood AA levels were measured at the end of the study, the older adults had markedly higher blood concentrations of AA.

This may explain, in part, why we see so much inflammation in the elderly, in the form of diseases like osteoarthritis. And it highlights yet another reason it is so vitally important for all of us to think preventively about these diseases, and to eat accordingly. We are so close to the line of overactive inflammation that we may move over that line, simply by the natural process of aging. Since we clearly can't control the aging process, it becomes even more important for us to control what we can: in this case, our diets.

> Controlling the amount of AA that we eat becomes even *more* important as we age.

This book was written to answer two fundamental questions: What are the factors causing the epidemic of inflammatory disease in industrialized countries? And how can you, as an individual, take control of your own inflammatory condition?

The answer to both those questions becomes painfully clear when we start looking—as we will in the next chapter—at the amount of AA that we take in through our diets. The foods that all of us eat a great deal of in industrialized countries are chock-full of AA.

This, then, is the poisoned trough—and I believe we have to look no farther than our own dinner tables to uncover a major reason why inflammatory disease is so rampant in this country, and why more of us are struck down with every passing year. No wonder, given the high level of AA in our diets, that the volume control on our immune systems is turned up to eleven, so that our immune systems launch full-scale attacks on healthy tissue and harmless invaders like pollen!

So our first step—and indeed, the first strategy in the Chilton Program—is to reduce the amount of AA we eat in our diets.

Chapter Six
Toxic Superfoods

As Joan scans her cookbook shelf for dinner ideas, she hears voices in the back of her head: her own family doctor warning against weight gain, now that her husband's arthritis has made their twice-weekly tennis game impossible; doctors on the news talking about essential fatty fish oils and Superfoods.

Beef stew and lamb chops are staples in her weeknight dinner rotation; she knows that the red meat has to go, although her mother's chicken dish can stay. She flips through the brightly colored pages of the cookbook until an easy recipe for Soy-Glazed Salmon catches her eye. Satisfied that she's helping her family take the first step toward good health, Joan jots down on her shopping list the ingredients she'll need.

Joan wants to do the best thing for her own health, and for the health of her husband. She's mindful of the health benefits of the omega-3 fatty acids, and she's concerned about cholesterol, so she's broadening her culinary horizons to include salmon. But Joan is so busy bailing out her boat with a tiny pail that she's blind to the iceberg up ahead. She would be horrified if she knew the truth: she's doing exactly the wrong thing. She's making that salmon dish in an effort to improve her husband's health, but instead, she may well be unknowingly contributing to his pain. If she sticks with their new regime, his days on the tennis courts may really and truly be over.

> Many of the foods we think are healthiest may actually be poisoning us.

If I accomplish one thing with this book, I want it to be the reversal of a devastating dietary trend: the consumption of "health" foods that are anything but.

In this chapter, we'll discover how the food we eat—including some of the foods we think are the very best choices for good health—is one of the forces playing a major role in driving the epidemic in inflammatory diseases.

The Superfood That May Be Making Us Sick

As Joan is about to learn, the foods we've been told are the most healthful may very well turn out to be truly hazardous for our overactive inflammatory systems.

Let's take her salmon dish as an example. Like many people, Joan has heard that salmon is one of the healthiest protein choices she can make. It contains high levels of two essential omega-3 fatty acids: eicosapentaenoic acid (EPA), and docosahexaenoic acid (DHA). These fatty acids have repeatedly been shown to have very positive health benefits, and I strongly believe they do. Diets high in these omega-3s have proven to lower blood pressure and triglyceride levels, to reduce platelet stickiness that can lead to heart attack and stroke, and even to impede the rapid growth of tumors.

If Joan's very savvy, she may even think that her choice of salmon will help her husband's arthritis. After all, EPA has been linked to relief from inflammatory diseases, including arthritis, for at least three decades. But Joan's in for a real surprise when we take a look at what's really hiding under that soy glaze.

Let's assume that the salmon she buys at her local supermarket or fish store is farmed, because most of the salmon available for sale in this country is. A four-ounce portion of farmed Atlantic salmon—less than the size of a standard filet—contains 1,306 milligrams of AA. That's more than *thirteen times* the amount of daily AA that I recommend in the Chilton Solution diet—or two weeks' worth! By choosing salmon for her family's dinner, Joan is dumping an enormous amount of AA right into their AA buckets, instead of the mere trickle that their bodies can actually handle—and that much AA can have important consequences for their health.

Let me put this in perspective for you by stealing that salmon off

Joan's plate and bringing it back into my own realm of scientific research. When researchers are proposing a study, their plans must be reviewed by an objective panel, called an institutional review board (IRB). This panel is designed to protect the human subjects involved in the study by ensuring their safety and ethical treatment at the hands of the researchers. Obviously, we're not in the business of endangering human lives in the name of scientific endeavor; you can't, for instance, poison people, or expose them to known carcinogens. The IRB is there to ensure that researchers can't and don't do anything that puts people participating in clinical studies at risk.

I don't believe there is an institutional review board in the country that would permit a long-term (several months or years) study that involved a daily level of AA comparable to the amount you'd find in a farmed Atlantic salmon steak.

While AA has been given in human studies at high concentrations for short periods of time, I cannot imagine designing a study that featured high concentrations of AA for any substantial amount of time. I don't believe there is an institutional review board in the country that would permit a long-term (several months or years) study that involved a daily level of AA comparable to the amount you'd find in a farmed Atlantic salmon steak.

You heard me right. It's considered sound medical practice to recommend at least two (and more, if possible) meals of fatty fish a week. And yet, I don't believe that a responsible medical review board would allow researchers to give on a daily basis, for more than a few weeks, the amount of AA in Joan's salmon to people participating in a study. The danger would simply be deemed too high.

This isn't just a pie-in-the-sky (or salmon en croute) fantasy. In 1975, a group of researchers at Vanderbilt University did just that. They introduced very high levels of arachidonic acid (several times the amount contained in a serving of farmed Atlantic salmon) into the diets of four study participants, in the form of a supplement, for twenty-one days, a relatively short period of time for a study.

As expected, this diet rapidly resulted in a dramatic increase in inflammatory messengers. That wasn't the only scary result. After just two weeks, researchers saw that the participants had dramatic increases in irreversible platelet aggregation, a leading contributor to heart attack. Because this was viewed as a substantive danger to two of the four participants, they were removed from the study.

So I believe a long-term experiment featuring a potentially hazardous amount of this fatty acid would be quashed for safety reasons before it even got off the ground. And yet we're happily sitting down to a salmon steak containing more than 1,300 milligrams of this inflammatory omega-6 fatty acid at Sunday dinner, poached and served with a dill sauce.

The Salmon Paradox

You'll note that I assumed that Joan's dinner was farmed salmon, not wild. This is a *critically important* detail. I made the assumption because most of the fish available for sale in this country is farmed. But wild salmon is available, and choosing it makes an enormous difference from the point of view of inflammation. While farmed salmon has astronomically high levels of AA, a similar portion of wild salmon has much less.

Compare the numbers yourself. According to the USDA, a four-ounce portion of farmed Atlantic salmon contains 1,306 milligrams of AA. The same-sized piece of wild Atlantic salmon has only 303 milligrams of AA—less than a quarter the amount. A four-ounce portion of wild Chinook salmon has 175 milligrams of AA, approximately seven times less.

> Farmed salmon has astronomically high levels of AA; a similar portion of wild salmon has much less.

How can salmon be so very, very good for you when it's wild, and so very bad for you when it's not?

For any fish, there are three major principles dictating its final fatty-acid composition. The first is the genetic capacity of that fish to transform the fatty acids that it consumes in its diet to other, highly unsaturated fatty acids such as AA or EPA. The second factor is the fish's diet: as the old saying goes, you are what you eat. The third factor is where that fish is raised. In general, fish raised in cold water have much more EPA and much less AA than fish raised in warmer waters.

To better understand the first two principles, let's go back to our "hole in the bucket" analogy. Human beings aren't very good at converting LA

Comparing Fatty Acids in Wild and Farmed Salmon

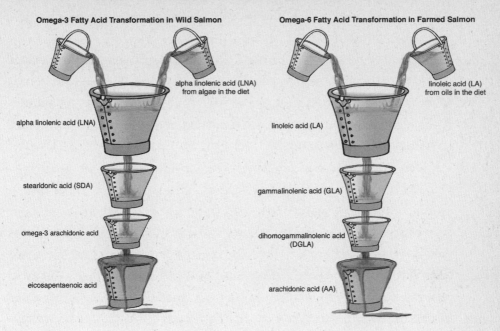

Omega-3 Fatty Acid Transformation in Wild Salmon | Omega-6 Fatty Acid Transformation in Farmed Salmon

alpha linolenic acid (LNA) from algae in the diet

linoleic acid (LA) from oils in the diet

alpha linolenic acid (LNA)

linoleic acid (LA)

stearidonic acid (SDA)

gammalinolenic acid (GLA)

omega-3 arachidonic acid

dihomogammalinolenic acid (DGLA)

eicosapentaenoic acid

arachidonic acid (AA)

into AA; our bodies limit these conversions, so they go very slowly. This means that the fatty acids leave our buckets in a slow trickle.

You may remember I mentioned that mice were better at these conversions. Salmon (and most other fish) are even better than mice. These fish are *extraordinarily* efficient at all of these fatty-acid conversions—they're like little factories in their ability to generate one fatty acid from another. Instead of the pinholes we found at the bottom of the human buckets, fish have great big holes, and the conversions go fast and furious as a result.

So salmon are very efficient at converting whatever fatty acids they eat into other fatty acids. This means that *what* they eat matters a great deal. Wild salmon eat primarily algae, which is wonderfully rich in omega-3 fatty acids that can be converted into those heart- and inflammatory-healthy omega-3s, EPA and DHA. Because they're so good at these conversions, wild salmon become rich sources of those fatty acids for the humans that eat them.

Farmed salmon, on the other hand, eat what they're fed, and that tends to be more omega-6 fats like the ones found in soybean and corn oil. In many cases, aquaculture, or the practice of fish farming, places enormous amounts of LA into the top bucket of those salmon. In humans, eating lots of LA isn't such a big deal, because, as we discussed, we aren't good at turning LA into AA. But because the salmon are so very good at moving those fatty acids through those conversions, when salmon eat a lot of LA, a great deal of AA ends up in that last bucket. And, of course, when we eat that AA-loaded salmon, we end up with lots of AA in our own buckets.

Joan might find the following piece of news even more upsetting: while fatty fish like mackerel and salmon are a rich source of the heart- and inflammatory-healthy fatty acids EPA and DHA, the farmed varieties contain considerably *lower* ratios of EPA and DHA to AA than the wild ones. In the example above, four ounces of the farmed salmon contains 700 mgs of beneficial EPA, while the wild Chinook salmon has 893. So in addition to getting huge levels of AA, Joan's not even balancing the health benefits of this AA with the beneficial EPA or DHA that she thought she was getting.

It's important to point out that I'm not against aquaculture, per se. Clearly, this industry arose at a time when our waters were overfished and there was an acute need for more fish. It's also important to note that not all fish farming results in "bad" fish. For example, according to the USDA, wild oysters contain more AA than farmed ones (they also contain more EPA). There are even circumstances where the farmed fish have *better* fatty-acid characteristics than wild fish. For example, farmed rainbow trout contains 260 milligrams of EPA and 25 milligrams of AA. Wild rainbow trout has less of the good EPA (167 milligrams) and four times *more* AA (109 milligrams) per serving.

So the objective of this book is certainly not to dismiss aquaculture out of hand. My only interest is to zero in on those fish that are likely to be the most pro-inflammatory because they contain very high levels of AA, and those fish that are likely to be the least inflammatory because they contain high levels of omega-3 fatty acids such as EPA and DHA, and have low AA-to-EPA ratios.

Barking Up the Wrong Tree

In many ways, the "health" industry has done Americans a tremendous disservice.

They've been telling us that salmon in general is one of the healthiest protein choices—and, in so doing, I believe they've contributed to an epidemic of inflammatory disease.

In the meantime, they've raised a tremendous alarm about issues with much less of a direct impact on our health. You can't turn on the news without hearing about PCBs and mercury in the fish we eat, and there has been a revolution in the food industry to meet the astonishing demand for organic vegetables and free-range, hormone- and antibiotic-free meat.

Nobody wants less pollution in our water, cleaner beef, and safer pesticide use more than I do. I am, however, concerned that our single-minded focus on these problems has distracted us while the real culprit was right in front of our noses. It's as if a gang of thugs has driven a moving van right up to our back door and is systematically robbing us of everything we own, even while we're installing the best and most high-tech burglar alarm on the market.

Nearly 50 percent of the people in this country suffer from inflammatory disease, and yet we consume more than a million metric tons of farmed Atlantic salmon a year.

This is one of the primary reasons I'm writing this book. I can no longer stand by while cardiologists continue to recommend the "Inflammation Blue Plate Special" to someone with heart disease and already elevated levels of inflammation. We have to turn a close eye on the way we eat, and we have to change what's on our plates.

The Incredible Inflammatory Egg

While levels of AA are astronomically high in fish like farmed Atlantic salmon, salmon is far from the only scoundrel in the *Inflammation Nation* story.

No other food source has been as hotly contested by nutritionists as the egg. Once a major villain in the cholesterol debate, the egg is back in vogue, now that farmers are fortifying eggs with omega-3 fatty acids by feeding the chickens flaxmeal and vitamin E, an antioxidant.

The inflammatory question, of course, has been left out of the debate. Eggs are one of the most significant sources of AA in our diets, with very little of the beneficial fatty acids to correct the balance. For example, two fried eggs contain 141 milligrams of AA and only 4 milligrams of EPA. Three scrambled eggs contain more than 200 milligrams of AA. And those are just the eggs you know about! Eggs are a "stealth ingredient." They appear—often without our knowledge—in many of the foods that we eat, from noodles to pancakes to baked goods to mayonnaise—and may be ratcheting up our inflammatory systems as a result.

Does fortification with omega-3 fatty acids reduce the inflammatory nature of the egg? It helps to some degree, but it is not a cure-all. While the amount of omega-3 fatty acids in eggs can be increased several times by feeding chickens omega-3 fatty acids, most studies show that omega-6 fatty acids (such as the inflammatory AA) are still at least as abundant as the omega-3s in these fortified eggs. In other words, no matter how much better these eggs are said to be, AA-to-EPA ratios still need to be improved.

If you look through the meal plans in this book, you'll see that you can eat eggs as long as you stick to just the whites, or to an egg substitute made primarily of egg whites. The high concentration of AA is in the yolk—and it's in the yolk of the egg where we can find an answer to one of the burning questions raised by our discovery of the connection between AA and inflammatory disease.

We know that there's more AA than there should be in some foods, like farmed salmon, because of changes in the way that food is produced—but *all* these foods, even in their most natural state, contain some AA. *If AA is so very bad for us, why is it present at all in our food?*

Enter the yolk. What, after all, is the purpose of an egg yolk, other than to appear sunny-side up on your breakfast plate? It's a food reserve for an embryonic chick. It turns out that babies—of all species—appear to need relatively high quantities of AA.

AA and DHA (docosahexaenoic acid) are important components of the central nervous system. These fatty acids are found in particularly high concentrations in the brain and retina of the eye, which would seem to suggest that they play an important role in the development of those very important organs. Recent studies have examined this combination in infants. Four hundred and seventy infants born prematurely were fed formulas with or without AA and DHA for one year. Eyesight, motor skills, and language abilities improved in the AA/DHA-supplemented group. By contrast, in full-term infants, AA/DHA had no impact on maturity levels.

These studies have made an impact on the marketplace in two important ways. The first is that formula companies began supplementing their products with AA and DHA. And studies such as these in preemies have led the dietary-supplement industry to create AA/DHA products for adults! While I believe that there are a number of benefits to taking DHA alone, I feel—for all the reasons set out in this book—that it would be a great mistake for adults to consume high concentrations of AA, unless there was proof that they were AA deficient.

Other Dietary Sources of Preformed AA

Some types of farmed fish and eggs are high in AA, but they're not the only things we're eating to make ourselves sick. Some of the livestock staples of the American diet also contain relatively high amounts of AA.

In almost all animals, organ tissues have higher amounts of AA than other tissues. For example, the concentration of AA in liver ranges from 120 milligrams to 250 milligrams per 100 grams, depending on the animal from which it is derived (see the Inflammatory Index in chapter 13). Other organ tissues including the heart, brain, and intestines also contain very high levels of AA.

In nonorgan tissues, the surfeit of preformed AA in livestock is the direct result of the market demands that have come about as a result of industrialization. Domestic animals are bred and raised to have a *vastly higher fat content* than those in the wild. Consider this: a wild pig contains about 1 percent to 3 percent fat. His domestic counterpart? Between 38 percent and 46 percent. A buffalo's fat percentage is also about 3 per-

Arachidonic Acid Content of Lean and Visible Fat in Meats

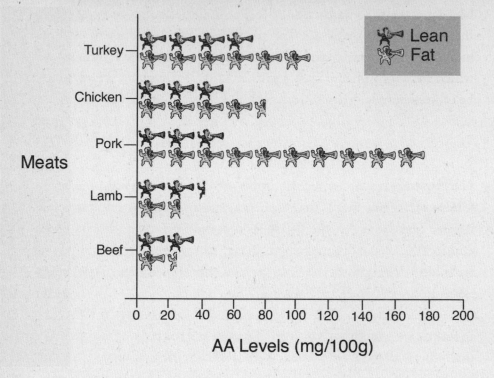

cent—but domestic beef weighs in at somewhere between 25 percent and 35 percent.

This makes a dramatic difference in the fatty-acid composition of the meats we get from these animals. In 1998, Dr. Andrew Sinclair published the most definitive study on AA concentrations in lean and fat animal tissues to date. (This study was done using Australian livestock, but we have no reason to believe that these numbers would be substantially different for animals raised in other developed countries.) Sinclair's study looked at AA amounts in beef, lamb, pork, chicken, and turkey. The highest level of AA in lean meat was in turkey. Pork fat took the prize for the fatty meat. There are about 50 milligrams of AA in lean pork; the same-sized portion of fatty pork contains three times as much AA, or about 170 milligrams.

Over the last thirty years, it's become commonplace for people to restrict their red meat consumption because of concerns about cholesterol. But for reasons we don't completely understand, beef and lamb are comparatively low in AA (as long as you stay away from organ tissues), and beef fat actually contains slightly less AA than the lean meat does. Dr. Sinclair and his colleagues also showed that lean beef and lamb contained higher levels of beneficial omega-3 fatty acids than the white meats, which were high in AA. Turkey, traditionally considered to be one of the healthiest choices, contains relatively high amounts of AA.

"No Thanks, I'm Watching My AA"

Curbing the amount of AA that we eat is one of the ways that the Chilton Program is able to stop out-of-control inflammation before it begins. The dietary model that I propose in order to bring our out-of-control AA levels back into check is very like another dietary model that has successfully made its way into the mainstream American consciousness: the low-cholesterol diet.

As with cholesterol, a certain amount of AA is essential for our body to function normally. But again, as with cholesterol, too much of this naturally occurring substance can lead to debilitating disease. Now, not everyone with heart disease has high cholesterol; similarly, not everyone with an inflammatory disease has elevated levels of AA and the inflammatory messengers it produces. But a large proportion of people are prone to converting dietary cholesterol to the artery-clogging kind—we call these people diet responders, because they can dramatically impact their health simply by changing their diets. When the steak and eggs stop, their cholesterol (and their risk of heart disease) drops.

The gathering scientific evidence indicates that there is a similar phenomenon in people who are particularly efficient at translating dietary AA into the overactive messengers behind inflammatory disease. When they limit their consumption of foods that contain high levels of AA, they produce much fewer of the messengers that cause inflammatory disease.

One of the very first lines of attack when we're tackling a high cholesterol problem is to reduce the

When inflammation sufferers restrict the amount of AA in their diets, they see a reduction in inflammatory messengers .

amount of cholesterol in the diet—*and the same thing should be true for AA*.
One day, I believe it will be commonplace for people to lower their AA
levels by restricting their AA intake, the same way it's now ordinary to
hear people ordering the heart-smart, low-cholesterol entrée in order to
improve their cholesterol levels.

I feel that this simple dietary solution will provide dramatic health
benefits, both for people living with debilitating chronic inflammatory
disease and for everyone else whose modern-day dietary habits are putting them at risk; these incredibly high stakes are why I feel that this book
is so very important right now.

The Plot Thickens

Clearly, those of us in industrialized societies are eating far too much AA,
with what I believe to be calamitous results for our immune systems,
which spin in overdrive because we're producing too many inflammatory
messengers.

AA isn't the only fatty acid we've thrown out of balance as a result of
the way we're now eating in industrialized nations. Remember, I prom-
ised you "a whole new look at fats," and I intend to deliver it.

Although AA is the central fatty acid governing the creation of a critical set of inflammatory messengers, it's not the only
fat with an effect on our inflammatory system. In
fact, there's a great deal of strong evidence to suggest that two other fatty acids—the omega-3
fatty acid called EPA and the omega-6 called
DGLA—play major roles as well.

> There are almost eight thousand articles in the scientific literature of the last thirty years linking fatty acids to inflammation.

You probably know that one of these essential
fatty acids, EPA, is vital to heart health, as Joan did.
This may not be the only benefit it brings. EPA and
DGLA work in tandem to act as inflammation fighters, by helping to
block the production of inflammatory messengers from AA, as well as
another category of inflammatory messengers called cytokines. I guess
you won't be too surprised to discover that these fatty acids are much

more prevalent in the diets of people in less-industrialized countries, and that they're very scarce in our own.

Veggie Delight

Although the anti-inflammatory properties of these essential fatty acids have taken a backseat to the promise they extend to those at risk for heart disease, these fatty acids have spent some time in the media spotlight. But the focus on these fatty acids has unwittingly given way to another huge and potentially damaging misconception: that the benefits conferred by these essential fatty acids can also be found from plant omega-3 fatty acids, such as the ones found in flaxseeds and flaxseed oil.

Flaxseed contains the omega-3 fatty acid alpha-linolenic acid. (Sorry. This sounds like, but *isn't*, linoleic acid or any of the fatty acids we've discussed previously in this chapter. For clarity's sake, we'll call it LNA.) The benefits of LNA and flaxseed oil have dominated the literature of the health-food industry, especially those that emphasize a vegetarian lifestyle. I wish I could tell you that I thought the LNA in flaxseed oil could replace wild fish as a rich source of the long-chain omega-3s like EPA and DHA, but the scientific literature simply does not support this contention.

Let's go back to our buckets. As we discussed, unlike mice and salmon, humans aren't very good at certain fatty-acid conversions. We're especially bad at some of them, including the conversion of LNA (the primary fatty acid in flaxseed oil) to the heart- and inflammatory-healthy omega-3s, EPA and DHA. We do the conversion, but very slowly, with the result that not much of those heart-healthy fatty acids get made. We also eat a lot of fatty acids (such as LA) that "compete" for enzymes that convert LNA to EPA and DHA, further limiting its conversion.

Consequently, although many reputable books (including some by doctors!) contend that flax is a viable, vegetarian alternative to fish oils, this is simply not the case. Flaxseed oil cannot replace wild fish as a source of omega-3s. I am particularly concerned about this assumption as it per-tains to children who are being raised as vegetarians. Many parents have been misled to believe that flaxseed oil can replace the essential fatty acids found in fish. In fact, it does not, and so these children may be short-changed of the foundational foods that their brains and bodies need to develop.

Is flax a better source of the essential fatty acids you need than, say, soybean oil? Yes, of course it is. But it cannot replace the fatty acids you get from eating wild fish, or taking a supplement derived from fish.

Does that mean that vegetarians have to swallow their principles, or condemn themselves to a life of inflammation and heart disease? Probably not. There are exciting new developments in this area entering the marketplace right now, in the form of plant seed oils with health benefits that may, to some degree, replace wild fish.

For example, there is a relatively new seed oil from a member of the borage family called *Echium plantagineum* (also known as Patterson's curse, dwarf blue bedder, or salvation Jane). This plant contains relatively high amounts of a fatty acid called stearidonic acid. Our laboratory has very recently demonstrated that this fatty acid is readily converted to heart- and inflammatory-healthy EPA—in other words, the fatty-acid conversions that humans happen to do well are the ones that transform stearidonic acid into EPA. Consequently, providing humans with stearidonic acid leads to significant quantities of EPA, the major fatty acid found in fish oil.

> Flaxseed oil cannot replace wild fish as a source of anti-inflammatory and heart-healthy fatty acids.

This means that, although it's a vegetable oil, stearidonic acid (SDA) may have many of the benefits of EPA. In fact, one of the most exciting results of the study we've just conducted showed a dramatic lowering of triglycerides in people with high levels. About 70 percent of the people in the study responded to the plant oil, and their response was notable: a 30 percent reduction in triglycerides. This triglyceride-lowering effect is one of the factors that make EPA so very good for your heart, which further strengthens the connection between stearidonic acid and EPA. I believe that seed oils such as echium will in the future play a very important role in human health.

A Culprit Exposed

A great deal of data now reveals that high levels of AA in the traditional Western diet is one of the major driving forces of the inflammatory epidemic sweeping America. It's ironic that some of the most dangerous foods—like farmed Atlantic salmon—are foods we consider to be among our healthiest choices. In short, our industrialized diet means that we're eating *more* of the fatty acids that increase inflammation and *not enough* of the ones that fight it.

We'll discuss these fats, and the mechanism by which they fight inflammation, in much greater detail when I show you the nuts and bolts behind the Chilton Program, but I can assure you that hope is in sight.

The Chilton Program rights the imbalance that contributes to inflammation by presenting you with a cohesive program that takes the correct proportions of these fatty acids into account. If you use the Inflammation Index that I've prepared especially for this book, you'll be eating fats in the correct ratios, and your body will be able to process them properly, instead of turning them into ammunition against itself. For the first time, you'll be able to attack inflammation before it starts. And I'll show you how, with a few painless changes to your diet, you'll start to bring your own overactive inflammatory system back into balance.

> We eat *too many* of the fatty acids that increase inflammation, and *not enough* of the ones that fight it.

PART 2

The Chilton Program

Chapter Seven
Bringing Overactive Inflammation Back into Balance

There's no doubt that development and industrialization have brought wonderful benefits into our lives—little things like indoor plumbing, advanced medical treatment, and the all-night corner store, just to name a few.

But as we know, industrialization has also radically changed our food supply. Let me give you an example. My neighbor usually considers his green thumb a blessing—until July, when the zucchini attack. He tries to give them away, but we hide when we see him coming. He and his wife make zucchini muffins, zucchini bread, zucchini quiche, zucchini chutney, pickled zucchini, zucchini carpaccio. There's zucchini in their stir-frys, their pasta dishes, their frittatas.

This seasonal abundance is the way we ate before trains, ships, and automobiles made it possible to buy the cornucopia of variety that awaits us in any American grocery store. Industrialization has radically changed the way we eat. Now, tomatoes from the Netherlands, avocados from Mexico, pears from Chile, cantaloupes from Arizona, and strawberries from California are no farther away than aisle six.

A wide variety of fruits and vegetables can be only a good thing, but the increased availability of certain kinds of carbohydrates and fats that have come with industrialization—specifically with the much wider availability of meat, eggs, and dairy—have had a much more negative impact on our health. I don't believe we are eating the foods we were designed to eat. As a direct result, our immune systems are turning against our bodies.

> I don't believe we are eating the foods we were designed to eat.

The Chilton Program is designed to correct the discrepancy between what we're supposed to be eating and what we actually eat, using a three-pronged strategy. Each component of the program isolates and corrects one of the systemic imbalances that has given rise to the out-of-control inflammation that's sweeping our individual bodies, as well as the nation as a whole. Three defenses are better than one, and together, I believe they are our best shot to reduce this epidemic. In this chapter, I'll walk you through the program, explaining the science behind each.

In part 3 of this book, I will give you the tools you need to eat healthfully for the rest of your life, but without complex calculations. Those tools include a food pyramid to replace the USDA's carbohydrate-heavy one; a fish chart, so you can ascertain your best and worst choices at a glance; and a revolutionary Inflammatory Quotient (IQ) quiz, which will tell you the inflammatory potential of any food.

By the time you've learned to use those tools, and have followed one of the two four-week meal plans provided, you will have learned a whole new way of eating: one in which food becomes a powerful tool to reduce—not worsen, as it does now—inflammatory diseases such as arthritis, asthma, inflammatory bowel disease, eczema, and atherosclerosis.

Step #1: Limit Arachidonic Acid

As described throughout this book, the inflammatory omega-6 fatty acid called arachidonic acid (AA) is one of the major building blocks for inflammatory messengers.

We obtain AA in our bodies one of two ways: from eating fatty acids in foods that can be converted to AA, or from eating foods that contain preformed AA. As you now know, humans don't do a good job of converting other fatty acids obtained from foods to AA, so we don't need to worry about that one. We *do* need to worry about the second. We *do* eat foods that contain preformed AA, and we eat them in great quantities, including dramatically high levels in some of the foods we consider to be healthiest, like salmon and eggs.

I believe we eat AA to our great detriment. Compelling evidence outlined in detail in chapters 5 and 6 makes it clear that the more AA we eat in our diets, the more messengers that cause inflammatory diseases we produce. High levels of AA in our bloodstream also lead to the production of messengers that cause platelet stickiness, a major risk factor for a heart attack, and patients who already have certain genetic markers leading to heart disease see their disease markedly worsen when they eat a lot of AA.

To make matters worse, the older we get, the more AA we accumulate in our blood, which may explain why inflammatory diseases are so common among older people. Other links between high levels of AA in our diet and our poor health are being discovered every day, and I suspect that this will remain a very fruitful area of research in the future.

Thus, I believe that one of the major factors fueling the inflammatory epidemic is the high levels of preformed AA that we consume in our diets.

And yet, the amount of AA that we eat has largely been ignored by the medical community. When I tell people about my work and explain the evidence for my dietary program, they almost invariably have the following reaction: "No offense, Dr. Chilton, but how come you're the first guy to think of this?" I wish I had an answer for that question. Certainly, the vast majority of the research money going into this field has focused on developing medications. That has greatly benefited people who suffer from these debilitating diseases, but it may explain why there hasn't yet been a dietary program that focused on avoiding preformed AA in our foods.

The evidence is clear: reducing the amount of AA we eat is one of the most direct ways to inhibit our body's ability to produce the inflammatory messengers that contribute to diseases such as arthritis, asthma, allergies, eczema, inflammatory bowel disease, and heart disease. Think of AA as the bullets in the gun. If you remove the bullets, the gun is rendered harmless.

But the amount of preformed AA in the typical American diet has *increased* steadily because of the changes that industrialization has wrought on our food supply. As outlined in chapter 6, we eat more of certain types of meats and eggs from domesticated livestock than we used to, and in greater portions, because industrialization has made those foods widely available and inexpensive. These foods contain large amounts of preformed AA.

Additionally, a large proportion of the fish we eat comes from fish farms. Some of these farm-raised fish (farmed Atlantic salmon, in particular) are given foods that turn them into dietary missiles, delivering dangerous levels of AA directly into our bodies when we eat them. Our first step, then, to combat out-of-control inflammation is to reduce the amount of AA that enters our bloodstream by controlling the amount of preformed AA we consume in our diets.

> Our first step to combat out-of-control inflammation is to reduce the amount of AA we eat.

In the same way that a person with high cholesterol can reduce his or her risk of heart attack by limiting the amount of dietary cholesterol consumed, I believe people with high levels of blood AA and out-of-control inflammation should restrict their dietary AA intake. By cutting the amount of AA that we eat, we're removing some of the building blocks that your body uses to create inappropriate amounts of inflammatory messengers.

Of course, these inflammatory messengers are important when produced in the proper amounts. You need to be able to protect yourself against real invaders, like opportunistic infection and bacteria. I want your body to have enough AA so that it can make the inflammatory messengers it needs—it's no victory if our efforts leave your body defenseless. So we're not taking *all* the bullets out of the gun. But reducing the quantity of those inflammatory messengers greatly inhibits the number of *inappropriate* responses—the full-bore attacks on our body's own tissue, or harmless invaders like pollen—that characterize inflammatory disease.

Step #2: Block the Critical Enzymes That Convert AA to Inflammatory Messengers

Limiting our dietary intake of preformed AA is the first dietary step toward bringing our overactive inflammatory systems back under control. While reducing your intake of dietary AA removes many of the bullets from the gun, it is next to impossible to remove enough AA from your diet to totally prevent the overproduction of inflammatory messengers, given our highly domesticated and processed food supply.

As described in chapter 4, AA doesn't automatically change into inflammatory messengers; it requires enzymes to do it. Enzymes are the keys that turn a chemical lock, like the heat under the pot that transforms tomatoes, onions, garlic, and some oregano into your grandmother's marinara sauce. Increasing the consumption of certain fatty acids (other than AA) actually blocks the ability of certain enzymes to convert AA to inflammatory messengers. Numerous studies, including many from my own laboratory, indicate that this approach has powerful anti-inflammatory benefits.

> The next step in the Chilton Program is to prevent important enzymes in our body from transforming AA into inflammatory messengers.

Thus, the second step in the Chilton Program is to make sure we're eating the proper amounts *and ratios* of the fatty acids that block the enzymes that convert AA to inflammation messengers.

As you'll remember, the omega-6s are—unfairly—labeled as the bad guys in today's popular dietary literature. While it is true that that we in developed countries are prone to eat way too much of many of the omega-6 fatty acids (including AA), creating high omega-6 to omega-3 ratios, it's important to remember that all omega-6s aren't created equal.

In particular, one member of the omega-6 family has been shown to be an extremely important *blocker* of that billion-dollar AA Pathway, preventing the production of the messengers that cause inflammatory diseases. So, contrary to the popular wisdom, indiscriminately cutting omega-6s may be doing you more harm than good. And, in fact, it was precisely *because* my team was so conditioned to think of the omega-6s as bad guys that it took us so long to recognize the potentially beneficial attributes of this one omega-6.

This "good" omega-6 fatty acid, the one that helps our bodies block the conversion of AA to inflammatory messengers, is dihomogammalinolenic acid (DGLA). Now, if you've already flipped through the Chilton Program, which appears a little later in this book, you may be wondering why I don't recommend that you take DGLA itself.

The answer to that question is that DGLA isn't available in significant quantities in our food supply, dietary supplements, or medical foods. If it were, you can be certain that I would be recommending it. So how do we get around this problem? This requires that we return to our "hole in the bucket" analogy (see figure on page 79 in chapter 5).

Since DGLA isn't available from food, we must ingest a fatty acid our bodies can turn into DGLA. That fatty acid is called gammalinolenic acid (GLA). My laboratory has shown that when we ingest GLA, inflammatory cells will take it up and rapidly convert it into DGLA. This leads to the accumulation of a natural—and very powerful—inhibitor of enzymes that convert AA to inflammatory messengers.

I recommend that you take GLA in the form of a supplement, instead of relying on food sources for it, because GLA has largely disappeared from our modern-day food supply. There's quite a bit of GLA in some nuts and seeds, which may explain why our bodies evolved with such a dependency on this fatty acid—as hunter-gatherers, we ate much larger quantities of nuts than we do now. In fact, according to S. Boyd Eaton, one of the foremost authorities on the Paleolithic diet, fruits, nuts, legumes, roots, and other noncereals provided 65 to 70 percent of the typical hunter-gatherer diet.

However, since the level of GLA you need to combat overactive inflammation is quite high, a handful of nuts or seeds won't do it. This fatty acid is readily available in capsule form at health food and supplement stores. GLA is found in many types of seeds and their oils, including borage, black currant, and evening primrose, and in pine nuts. Borage seed is an ideal source of GLA, because more than 20 percent of the fatty acids in the seed oil is GLA. Borage was originally cultivated in Syria. It was a favorite with the ancient Romans, who used it to flavor their wines and beers. Today, several companies are attempting to put this oil and other GLA-containing oils into foods.

Much of my initial interest in the anti-inflammatory effects of GLA arose from a pivotal study carried out by Robert Zurier, which was published in the *Annals of Internal Medicine* in 1993. In this rigorous, placebo-controlled, twenty-four-week trial, Dr. Zurier's group demonstrated that high doses of GLA caused marked reductions in the number of, and in the pain from, tender joints in patients with rheumatoid arthritis. The placebo group did not show significant improvement in any of these measures. The study concluded, "GLA, in doses used in this study, is a well-tolerated and effective treatment for active rheumatoid arthritis." Subsequent studies found similar results. So, there is science-based, clinical evidence that GLA, under the right conditions, can be a powerful and natural anti-inflammatory agent.

You may have heard about GLA discussed in inflammatory disease circles; formulations of this supplement are already marketed as anti-inflammatories, largely because of the study cited above (as well as some other, less rigorous ones). You may even have tried some of these supplements without success. This time will be radically different. For the past decade, my laboratory carried out its own studies to understand just how GLA has these powerful anti-inflammatory effects. These studies, published in five peer-reviewed scientific journals, demonstrate that critical inflammatory cells gobble up dietary GLA and rapidly transform it into DGLA, which efficiently and naturally reduces the formation of inflammatory messengers.

While several studies attempted to unravel the connection between this supplement and inflammation, my laboratory was the first to focus on how to use the supplement in a truly effective and safe manner. Why? Historically, patients, clinicians, and researchers have made two major mistakes when using GLA as a dietary supplement.

First, they have not used GLA in sufficiently high quantities to influence inflammatory messenger levels in the body. For example, my laboratory has shown that (depending on how it is given), at least 600 milligrams of GLA are required each day to have significant effects on the inflammatory messengers produced by our body. The typical 1 g capsule has about 200 milligrams of GLA, so you have to take three capsules a day to see an effect. If you've taken this supplement in doses too small to see results, please know that there's a silver lining to what must seem like wasted effort and money: taken by itself, GLA has a dangerous side effect that we'll discuss in a moment. When you read what I have to say, you may be very happy you weren't taking a large enough dose to make a difference.

How you take your daily supplement of GLA is also very important.

The data is clear that the fatty acids in these supplements make it through your digestive tract to the bloodstream much more efficiently if they are provided as a liquid emulsion or as gel capsules taken with food. When they're taken alone, a smaller proportion of fatty acids make it to your bloodstream. As you'll see, the menu plans in the Chilton Program will specifically prompt you to take your supplement so that you can make it a part of your daily eating routine to maximize its effectiveness.

In addition to underestimating the amount of GLA needed to reduce inflammatory messenger levels, researchers have traditionally made another, even more crucial mistake. If GLA is not provided with the right combination of fatty acids, it has a tricky side effect, one that must be sidestepped if we are going to take advantage of the anti-inflammatory effects of GLA.

As discussed above, inflammatory cells readily convert GLA into the very beneficial DGLA, so you can envision the GLA bucket delivering a steady stream of anti-inflammatory goodness into the DGLA bucket. But DGLA isn't the only fatty acid that can be formed from GLA. Stay with me on the science here: it's really just a different take on our old "bucket" analogy.

GLA is transformed into DGLA, but, as I just noted, that's not the only fatty acid it can form. In fact, GLA is actually delivering two separate streams into two different buckets. One stream represents the GLA in your diet that's delivered to your inflammatory cells; the other stream is the GLA that is delivered to your liver. The GLA that is delivered to your inflammatory cells is transformed into the inflammation-friendly DGLA. Unfortunately, the GLA that goes to your liver is converted to AA—the exact thing we're trying to avoid!

I remember the first time that I saw this result in my lab. You could have knocked me over with a feather, and not just because it was exactly the opposite result from the one I was hoping to find. At that moment, I realized that all those people who were already taking high amounts of GLA, presumably to help their inflammatory problems, were exposing themselves to extremely high levels of circulating AA.

That's not just a problem for the obvious reason, because too much AA causes an overabundance of the inflammatory messengers, but as you

The Two Paths of GLA Transformation

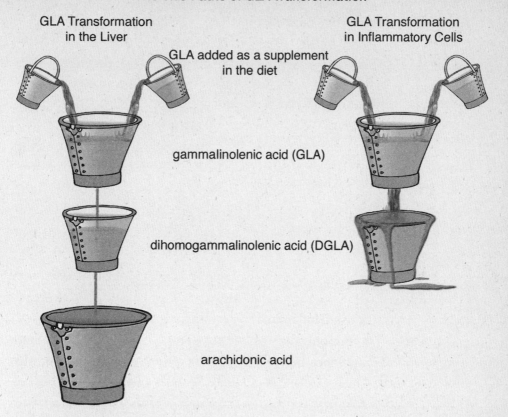

GLA Transformation
in the Liver

GLA Transformation
in Inflammatory Cells

GLA added as a supplement
in the diet

gammalinolenic acid (GLA)

dihomogammalinolenic acid (DGLA)

arachidonic acid

will remember from chapters 5 and 6, high levels of circulating AA can cause increased platelet stickiness, which is associated with cardiovascular events such as heart attacks. So taking too much GLA can actually put you at risk for a cardiac event. They don't tell you that at the health-food store!

Fortunately, my laboratory found a simple way around this problem: the conversion of GLA to AA by the liver can easily be blocked by increasing our consumption of another fatty acid, eicosapentaenoic acid (EPA), which is found in wild fish. If you are taking high levels of anti-inflammatory GLA, you *must* make sure you are getting enough EPA to block the potentially dangerous side effect of this powerful supplement.

So the third fatty acid in our cooldown equation,

> If you take high levels of GLA, you must also take EPA to block potentially dangerous side effects.

Then and Now: The Fatty Acid Difference

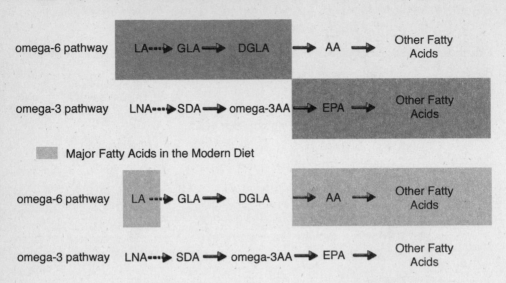

along with AA and GLA, is EPA. EPA blocks the body's ability to turn GLA into AA, an essential piece of the puzzle if we want to maintain the beneficial effects of GLA while eliminating the inadvertent side effect of increased AA, the very substance we're trying to curb.

This also makes a great deal of sense in terms of the hunter-gatherer diet. In addition to fruits, nuts, legumes, roots, and other noncereals, early man ate a great deal of shellfish, which contains high levels of EPA. That's why the hunter-gatherer diet is estimated to have had an omega-6 to omega-3 fatty-acid ratio of 1:1, as opposed to the ratio of 20:1 found in most American diets today. From an evolutionary perspective, it makes perfect sense that we'd need to have a combination of GLA and EPA for our immune systems to work properly.

Let me spell this out. Hunter-gatherers would have gotten the LA they needed from the animals they hunted for food; the GLA they needed from the nuts, legumes, and roots they gathered; the EPA from the shellfish they ate. Because the animals they ate were much lower in fat, as venison and other game meats are today, they would have gotten very little AA from their diets. In other words, hunter-gatherers were getting a near-perfect balance of polyunsaturated fatty acids for the optimal operation of their immune systems, simply by eating what was available to them. By contrast, the meat and fish we eat today are loaded with AA and LA, and we get very little GLA and EPA from our diets.

So, as you can see (literally, in the accompanying figure), we're eating a different balance—in fact, almost the complete *opposite* proportion—of the fatty acids our ancestors ate. They were getting a perfect balance, the balance our bodies are genetically designed to consume. Ours, tragically, is a much less favorable ratio.

My laboratory has carried out numerous studies and clinical trials to determine the precise amounts and ratios of GLA to EPA necessary to maximize the inhibition of inflammatory messengers without raising the level of AA in the blood. The great news is that this ratio is easily achieved when you combine a GLA supplement with the right foods, like wild fish, that contain both a small amounts of AA and a lot of EPA.

The health benefits of EPA are well reported, and many health-conscious people are already choosing fatty fish like salmon in an attempt to get more of these fatty acids into their diets. But again, what the aver-

Fatty Acids Added to Our Diets by the Chilton Program

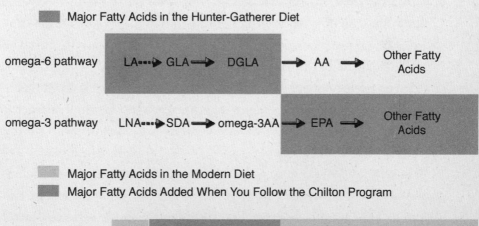

Major Fatty Acids in the Hunter-Gatherer Diet

| omega-6 pathway | LA····▶ GLA ➡ DGLA ➡ AA ➡ Other Fatty Acids |
| omega-3 pathway | LNA····▶SDA ➡ omega-3AA ➡ EPA ➡ Other Fatty Acids |

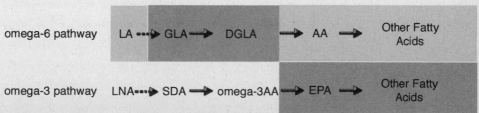

Major Fatty Acids in the Modern Diet
Major Fatty Acids Added When You Follow the Chilton Program

| omega-6 pathway | LA ····▶ GLA ➡ DGLA ➡ AA ➡ Other Fatty Acids |
| omega-3 pathway | LNA····▶ SDA ➡ omega-3AA ➡ EPA ➡ Other Fatty Acids |

age consumer *doesn't* know is that while wild fatty fish like mackerel and salmon are a rich source of EPA, farmed fish, like Atlantic salmon, contain considerably less of this beneficial fatty acid than the wild ones—and, more important, they contain potentially dangerous quantities of AA. So when you're sitting down to your heart-healthy salmon dinner, as many popular diets recommend, you're not only *not* getting the health benefits you bargained for, but you are potentially worsening an already bad situation!

As you can see from the figure on the previous page, the Chilton Program brings your polyunsaturated fatty acid ratio back into the balance your hunter-gatherer forebears got naturally from their diets. You'll get less AA, and more GLA and EPA—as they did. I'll also provide you with supplementation information, so that you get enough of these fatty acids no matter what you eat.

Step #3: Eat Carbohydrates with a Low-to-Moderate Value on the Glycemic Index

The Chilton Program delivers an optimal balance of three fatty acids that govern inflammation. But balancing fatty acids isn't the only way the Chilton Program douses the flames of inflammation. We also address another essential macronutrient, one that has come to the forefront of the nutritional debate in the last few years: the carbohydrate.

As you go through the diet plans included in this book, in some respects, you'll see that parts of my program share some common elements with other high-protein/lower-carbohydrate diet plans such as the Atkins and South Beach diets.

I respect both of these diets for the way they've taken on some dietary sacred cows and changed the way Americans think about nutrition. The Atkins diet challenged the prevailing view that all fats are bad and that all carbohydrates are good. The Mediterranean and South Beach diets, with their focus on reducing saturated fat, introduced the public to the idea that we have to get the *right* fats and carbohydrates in our diets for optimal cardiac health.

But these diets have taken us only part of the way up the mountain;

my eating program takes us to the next level by further refining *precisely* the types of fats and carbohydrates that should be included and avoided.

As you've already seen, I'm much more specific even than South Beach on the question of fats. Because inflammation wasn't taken into account in that diet, I found that many of the recommendations (like the emphasis on foods like salmon, with no differentiation between wild and farmed, and on eggs) were potentially dangerous from an inflammation perspective.

I've already made it clear why we need to be more specific about the way we choose our proteins and our fats. It's time to bring that same level of specificity to the kinds of carbohydrates we should be eating.

In the Chilton Program, you'll find the perfect inflammation-extinguishing ratio of the three fatty acids mentioned above, but you'll also find a strong emphasis on high-fiber, "whole" carbohydrates, like the ones found in fruits, vegetables, and whole grains. These carbohydrates, and others, like beans and legumes, dairy products, slow-cooking cereals, and whole-grain breads, receive a low-to-moderate score on the Glycemic Index. You will find a ranking that takes this index into account in chapter 14. This, then, is our third inflammation-fighting strategy. The final step of the Chilton Program focuses on stabilizing blood sugar by encouraging you to eat carbohydrates with a low-to-moderate value on the Glycemic Index.

> The final step of the Chilton Program: eat carbohydrates with a low-to-moderate value on the Glycemic Index.

The Glycemic Index is a measure of how rapidly carbohydrates break down and affect blood sugar. Refined, or white, carbohydrates (think white bread and table sugar) are digested rapidly; those sugars flood the bloodstream very quickly. These foods can make you fat and cause a myriad of diseases, including metabolic syndrome, or Syndrome X, and type 2 diabetes. By contrast, complex carbohydrates, like the ones found in vegetables and whole grains, are digested much more slowly; so the glucose and insulin are released into the bloodstream gradually. What, you might ask, does any of this have to

> High levels of glucose and insulin are linked to the production of inflammatory messengers from AA.

do with inflammation? Quite a lot, actually. Yes, refined carbohydrates are bad for you in all the ways that Atkins and South Beach told you they were, but it's not just your waistline you have to worry about, but the very real threat of inflammatory disease! Like fatty acids, choosing the right carbohydrates is essential, not just in the fight against obesity and related disorders, but in the battle against inflammation as well.

Here's why:

High levels of glucose and insulin are linked to the production of inflammatory messengers from AA.

There are several reasons for this. First of all, high levels of insulin activate enzymes that cause our body to make more AA. Second, insulin controls the conversion of AA to inflammatory messengers, leukotrienes and prostaglandins. This effect is not always predictable: at some concentrations, insulin actually inhibits inflammatory messenger production, while at others, it stimulates them. Third, inflammatory messengers from AA (both prostaglandins and leukotrienes) in turn regulate circulating insulin levels. In other words, insulin both regulates, and is regulated by, the inflammatory messengers of AA.

Finally, there is a newly discovered group of molecules, called PPARs (peroxisome proliferator-activated receptors), that controls glucose uptake. These molecules can be activated by certain dietary fatty acids such as AA, and a new class of inflammatory messengers made from AA. While the biochemistry of PPARs is beyond the scope of this book, this is an extremely important and exciting area of research that will greatly impact our understanding of glucose regulation in the near future.

So there's a complex interaction between messengers of inflammation, leukotrienes and prostaglandins, and insulin and glucose levels. It's not as simple as cause and effect, but we can say that there is a strong connection between blood sugar levels, the systems that control those levels, and inflammation. This means that there's an intimate relationship between inflammation and the kinds of carbohydrates we consume. Clearly, this relationship must be taken into account if we are to control inflammation.

Eating too many of the wrong kind of carbohydrates will sabotage the anti-inflammatory effect of this diet.

You'll want to avoid anything that dramatically

alters glucose and/or insulin levels, which is what happens on an hourly basis when you eat too many refined carbohydrates. These spikes and drops in blood sugar level make it practically impossible to control inflammatory messengers, no matter how perfect your fatty-acid ratios are, because we can't isolate the carbohydrate and fatty-acid systems from one another. They work together, in synergy, so following my third rule is absolutely essential if your goal is to curb inflammation. Eating too much of the wrong kind of carbohydrates will sabotage the anti-inflammatory effect of this diet.

As you'll see when you review the meal plans, sticking with foods ranked low to moderate on the Glycemic Index doesn't mean you're stuck on one of those scary, all-protein, deprivation diets. You absolutely don't have to—and shouldn't—deprive yourself of satisfying, delicious, fiber-and nutrient-packed foods such as black bean soup and sweet potatoes—you just have to choose the right ones. To make it simple for readers, *Inflammation Nation* includes an additional tool, a Glycemic Index ranking that lists foods grouped into high, moderate, and low categories; you'll easily be able to choose the best carbohydrates for you.

Another benefit of the carbohydrates with moderate-to-low rankings on the Glycemic Index is that they're high in fiber. Fiber is another major component in short supply in the American diet. Let's go back to our hunter-gatherer ancestors. It is estimated that they consumed more than a hundred different species of fruits and vegetables, providing more than 100 grams per day of fiber. According to the National Center for Health Statistics, people in the United States today average only 14 to 15 grams of fiber intake per day. That's a considerable discrepancy! But it's not surprising when you look at what we eat. In fact, it would be very difficult to design a diet, using foods from the standard American food supply, that contained anywhere near the amount of fiber that our hunter-gatherer ancestors consumed. That said, we can—and should—do better on fiber, so the Chilton Program contains an average of 30 grams of fiber per day.

And, as with the fatty acids in my program, you can even cheat a little. On my program, you won't have to say no to a slice of chocolate cake at your daughter's birthday party. Of course, you don't want to get into the habit of indulging every day. Not only will you negate the good inflammation-fighting work you're doing on the fatty-acid side, but the human body has a tendency to get "addicted" to a regular infusion of these refined carbs. However, the occasional treat won't hurt you, and it will make staying on this diet for the long run a great deal easier for you.

Summary

By lowering the amount of AA that you eat, you decrease the amount of AA in your bloodstream, reducing the number of building blocks your body has to produce inflammatory messengers. By taking in a more balanced ratio of GLA and EPA, you will enable your body to block the production of inflammatory messengers. And by choosing the right carbohydrates, ones low on the Glycemic Index, you will regulate the blood sugar systems that both affect, and are affected by, the inflammatory messengers.

Like the individual strands of a braided rope, the three steps of the Chilton Program work—together and apart—to reduce dramatically the overactive inflammation that causes inflammatory disease.

Chapter Eight

Your Anti-Inflammatory Arsenal

In order to have an impact on this epidemic of inflammatory diseases, and to provide some help and relief from symptoms for individual sufferers, we must change the way we eat. I believe that the dietary program outlined in this book can provide you with a better model for the food choices you make in the future so that you're using food to help your body protect itself against illness and disease, not as an instrument of harm.

This will require a shift in the way you think about food, which is more easily said than done. Our lives are busy and hectic. All too often, we make food choices based on what's most convenient, quickest, and cheapest, instead of what's healthiest. And, as I have said throughout this book, we are going to have to change our fundamental conception about what those healthiest foods are.

So I realize the magnitude of what I'm asking you to do here, and I have only this to offer in return: **you will feel better.** If you are already sick, clinical studies reveal that you will reduce inflammatory messengers that cause symptoms of your inflammatory disease in as few as seven days. And, whether you are already sick or not, by following the rules of my program, you will reap great preventative benefits from restoring your body's natural balance, lowering your overall level of inflammation, and heading off future disease at the pass.

Because I know it's hard to change eating habits, and because I know that this is a new way of thinking about inflammatory disease, I designed the Chilton Program to be as easy to adapt and integrate into your life as possible. I did this in a number of ways:

The Chilton Program uses ordinary foods. The foods used in this diet are ordinary American table foods. You don't have to learn to love some grain you've never heard of before, and you don't have to mail order any bizarre ingredients. You won't have to alter your diet beyond all recognition: chances are good that you can still eat most, if not all, of the foods you like.

You won't go hungry. The foods used in this diet are predominantly whole foods, with a concentration on fish, lean meats, vegetables, nuts, and healthy fats. These protein-rich, high-fiber foods have a high satiety factor, which is a fancy way of saying that they fill you up. I know one thing: if you're not full, you'll eventually cheat and eat until you are. It's only human.

I provide easy-to-use, at-a-glance tools. One of the consistent problems with the nutritional information disseminated in this country is how confusing it is. Dissenting voices call out from every corner, with the result that intelligent people can't tell how best to proceed. I've taken the guesswork out of anti-inflammatory eating with the tools we'll be discussing in this chapter. (You'll find the tools themselves in part 3 of this book.) These tools include the Inflammatory Index, which assigns each food a number, depending on its profile of inflammatory fatty acids; the Chilton Fish Ranking, so you can quickly ascertain your best and worst fish options; the Glycemic Index, which will help you to choose the best and worst carbohydrates; and the Chilton Pyramid, which presents your optimal food choices in a visual layout.

The Inflammatory Index

In order to help you manage your dietary intake of AA, I've devised a unique tool called the Inflammatory Index (page 165). I like to think of this index as the secret weapon of the Chilton Program: this simple, easy-to-read chart is designed to help you control your fatty-acid intake for optimum inflammatory health.

Since we've gotten very carb- and fat-conscious as a society, companies now include these values on the sides of packaged foods so that consumers can calculate their meals accordingly. Since the relevant fatty-acid values such as AA and EPA don't appear on those labels (just yet!), I've created the Inflammatory Index to allow you to evaluate—at a single glance—the inflammation potential of several foods based on their content of important fatty acids.

Avoiding preformed AA in our food is the first strategy of the Chilton Program. So I began with the first-ever database of AA values, taken from the USDA, and assigned foods a value depending on how great their concentration of AA is. As you'll remember, AA isn't the only fatty acid we're concerned about in food. We also wanted to take into consideration other fatty acids, such as EPA, which blocks the absorption of AA into inflammatory cells. So I took the Inflammatory Index one step further and took the concentration of EPA into account as well. Foods with a low—and therefore good—rating on the Inflammatory Index have either low concentrations of AA, or high concentrations of EPA and moderate concentrations of AA. You can see Appendix B for the equation used to come up with the values in the Inflammatory Index.

I did the calculations for some of the most common foods so that you don't have to, and you'll find the results in the Values column of the final Inflammatory Index. Now, for the first time, there is a tool that takes into consideration the precise ratio and concentration of fatty acids that have an impact on your inflammatory response.

> The Inflammatory Index gives every food an "inflammatory value."

The Inflammatory Index makes it easy to replace some of your less-healthy, pro-inflammatory food choices with other, less-inflammatory ones. All you have to do is choose foods with a low index value, and keep your overall daily values within the parameters of the diet—prevention or solution—that you're following. The Inflammatory Index will enable you to plan an endless array of tempting meals while keeping the amount of AA in your diet under control with just a quick glance, with no more effort than you already expend managing your calories and your carbs.

This isn't one of those all-or-nothing diets that people find so difficult to follow for any length of time—there's built-in flexibility to allow for individual choice. You can absolutely choose to eat a food that has a greater Inflammatory Index value, as long as your other food choices over the course of the day allow you to stay under your daily limit.

Better still, you can even cheat every once in a while! The diet is deliberately calibrated to work as long as you stay within the parameters the majority of the time. I've explained that it takes about two weeks for the benefits of this diet to wear off. That means that an occasional indulgence won't hurt you, which makes the overall diet plan much easier to stick with.

The Chilton Fish Ranking

Fish is one of the hot-button issues in this diet. On the one hand, fish is one of the healthiest protein choices we can make, because it's relatively low in calories and saturated fat, and rich in other nutrients, including omega-3 fatty acids that are so good for our hearts and have such stunning anti-inflammatory potential. On the other hand, I believe that certain fish, especially those that come from fish farms where they're fed large amounts of omega-6 fatty acids and become heavy-duty sources of AA, have played a significant role in the increase in inflammatory disease in this country. I believe that eating these fish can be injurious to our health.

On the Chilton Program, you'll be encouraged to eat more fish than you may be used to eating in your standard diet, but because all fish isn't created equal, we'll be focusing very closely on which fish to choose. The Chilton Fish Ranking (page 172) will show you—at a glance—your most anti-inflammatory choices, and which selections you should avoid.

WHAT IF YOU DON'T LIKE FISH?

I love fish, and I hope that this book encourages people to incorporate more fish into their diets. But I do understand that some people don't like fish, or don't want to eat it as often as I recommend.

If you don't like fish, you can still do the Chilton Program. You'll simply have to add an EPA supplement. These supplements are readily available at health-food stores. For more information about assuring the quality of the supplements you take, please see www.inflammationnation.com. For specific dosage information, please see recommendations for the Chilton Prevention Diet, starting on page 176, or the Chilton Solution Diet, starting on page 205.

Best Fish and Good Fish (Category 1 and 2)

The fish that are lowest in AA and highest in EPA receive my highest ranking: Best Fish. In the meal plans, these will be known as Category 1 fish. Fish with a slightly less beneficial ratio of AA to EPA receive a ranking of Good Fish, or Category 2, as they'll be known in the plans.

Fish in both of these categories count toward your daily EPA. If you do not eat a portion of one of these fish, I'd encourage you to take an EPA supplement to make up the difference. (For more information about supplementation, please see chapter 11.)

I would encourage you to add as many of these types of fish to your diet as possible. The meal plans should help to show you ways that you can incorporate them into your diet. This category includes fish like mackerel, some types of wild salmon, and halibut from Greenland.

Neutral Fish (Category 3)

The next category is Neutral Fish, and the name tells you everything you need to know. These fish aren't bad for you—their AA/EPA ratio isn't detrimental—but neither do they add fatty-acid value to your diet. In general, they just don't contain enough AA or EPA to be placed in any of the aforementioned categories. Thus, they're neutral.

Can you eat them? Yes. I would prefer to see you use those calories on fish that has a more positive impact on your inflammatory health, but if you find one of your favorites on this list, you can absolutely eat it. If you do choose these fish, I do encourage you to take an EPA supplement to make up for the fatty-acid benefit these fish do not provide. This list includes fish and some types of shellfish such as trout, swordfish, scallops, and mussels.

Bad Fish (Category 4)

I ordinarily shy away from black-and-white terminology like "good" and "bad" when I'm talking about foods, but I believe there are foods that people who suffer from inflammatory disease and people who are at high risk for these diseases should avoid. The fish on this list are some of those foods, including farmed Atlantic salmon, grouper, and halibut from the Atlantic or the Pacific. Fish make it to this category either because they have very high amounts of AA, or because their AA/EPA ratio is poor.

The Glycemic Index

Choosing the right carbohydrates is as important as choosing the right fatty acids when you do the Chilton Program. Because blood sugar and the hormones that regulate it have an impact on inflammatory messengers (and the other way around), it's in your best inflammatory interest to keep your blood sugar fairly stable. High levels of glucose and insulin are linked to the production of inflammatory messengers from AA, as well as with insulin resistance.

The Glycemic Index measures how rapidly carbohydrates break down and affect blood sugar. It is the gold standard used to measure the impact of carbohydrates on insulin levels, and it's one of the tools you'll be using in the Chilton Program in order to keep your insulin levels under control.

When you eat a piece of candy, it breaks down very fast into glucose, and the body has to make a lot of insulin to ferry that glucose into the cells for storage. Then there's too much insulin in the blood, and you "crash," feeling hungry, irritable, or fatigued until you eat more sugar, and the cycle starts again. By contrast, when you eat the kind of carbohydrate that breaks down more slowly—a bowl of brown rice and vegetables, for instance—the glucose created by their breakdown seeps slowly into the bloodstream instead of flooding it. As a result, the body's insulin production can be much more moderate, and the interaction between this hormone and inflammatory messengers is much more moderate as well.

If you don't control your insulin, you can't control your inflammatory levels.

In order to keep blood sugar and insulin levels within a healthy range, choose carbohydrates that are low-to-moderate on the Glycemic Index, the high-fiber, "whole" carbohydrates, like the ones found in vegetables, beans and legumes, dairy products, slow-cooking cereals and whole grains, some fruits, and whole-grain breads.

And, yes, you can sneak the occasional food that ranks high on the Glycemic Index, as long as you don't do it every day. Many people find that they're addicted to these foods, and that there is no such thing as "a little" cake, or just one cookie. Those people find it's easier just to cut these foods from their diets altogether. Once they've broken the stranglehold that these refined carbohydrates have on them, they find it much easier to pass the dessert plate—especially when they know how much better they feel.

The Chilton Pyramid

The USDA first released its Food Pyramid in 1992; by 1994, it appeared on many packaged foods. You're probably familiar with its recommendations: five to eleven servings from the bread, cereal, rice, and pasta group; three to five servings from the vegetable group; two to four servings from the fruit group; two to three servings from the milk, cheese, and yogurt group; two to three servings from the meat, poultry, fish, dry beans, and eggs group; and the caution to "use sparingly" of the fats, sweets, and oils group.

This pyramid has come under a lot of fire of late. Although it still appears on many packaged foods, there's pretty much a unanimous sentiment among doctors and nutritionists that the recommendations—brought about to reverse the high levels of heart disease in the American population—simply aren't working. Opponents have pointed out that a diet heavy in grains is precisely what farmers use to fatten cattle—so it's no wonder that obesity rates are skyrocketing, when the recommendations are so heavily weighted toward cereals and grains.

In fact, Atkins, the low-carbohydrate proponents, have gone so far as to issue their own food pyramid, which features protein sources (such as eggs, fish, tofu, and steak) on the bottom, "eat most often" level, followed by vegetables, then fruits, then oils from vegetables and seeds, cheese and dairy, nuts and legumes, with whole grains and whole-grain foods at the very top, in the "eat least often" category.

Even people who believe that a low-calorie, high-carbohydrate diet is the way to go for weight loss and optimal health object to the USDA

Food Pyramid's failure to differentiate between whole grains and their processed alternatives, or to make a distinction between meats heavy in saturated fats like prime rib, and the other protein sources such as fish or lentils.

Obviously, no one has looked at the USDA Food Pyramid (or the food pyramids of any of its detractors) for inflammatory potential. I, too, am disappointed to see that there is no differentiation made between whole carbohydrates and processed, refined ones. And obviously, no one has gotten quite as specific about the kinds of protein I recommend you eat—and those, like whole eggs, that I think you would be better off avoiding.

That said, I do think that a pyramid is an effective way to communicate what you can eat, and in what proportions. So I am pleased to present the Chilton Pyramid, below.

As you can see, the Chilton Program represents a significant departure from the previous pyramids you may have become familiar with. It

The Chilton Food Pyramid

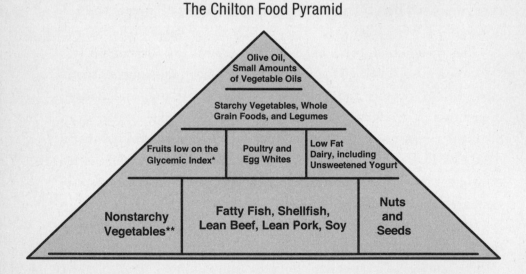

Eat sparingly from foods at the top of the pyramid, and more often from the ones at the base. Eat processed flour and refined sugars as rarely as possible.

* **Fruits low on the glycemic index** include: peaches, grapes, plums, strawberries, and grapefruit

** **Nonstarchy vegetables** include: lettuce, kale, broccoli, cucumber, spinach, mushrooms, tomatoes, green beans, cabbage, asparagus, and squash

emphasizes protein, but all proteins are not the same, because the fatty acids they deliver aren't the same. So the Chilton Program focuses on wild fish and lean meats. Unlike Atkins, which also focuses on protein, poultry plays less of a significant role in the Chilton Pyramid, and egg yolks play no role at all. I'm more specific about vegetables than the USDA Food Pyramid, and place the focus of my diet on nonstarchy vegetables, like broccoli and the lettuces.

I hope that the Chilton Pyramid—and the other tools presented in this book—are useful in helping you to make anti-inflammatory food decisions in the future.

The Chilton Program is a new way of thinking about inflammatory disease, and it's natural to have questions about the way this program will work to prevent, manage, and even reverse the overactive inflammation that gives rise to inflammatory disease.

I hope that the answers to some of the questions I've been asked most often will clear up your outstanding queries about the Chilton Program.

How will following the Chilton Program help me?

Here is what we know. Six clinical trials (with six peer-reviewed scientific journal publications) reveal that the fatty-acid balance in the Chilton Program blocks the production of inflammatory messengers that cause signs and symptoms of inflammatory diseases. Blocking these inflammatory messengers is a proven therapeutic approach for the management of inflammatory diseases.

Therefore, based on the science, I believe that I have designed a dietary program that will play a critical role in managing disease flares and, in some cases, preventing devastating inflammatory diseases in sufferers who add this diet program to their lives.

How long will the Chilton Program take to work?

Based on the science described above, I believe that you will begin to see relief from symptoms in as little as seven to ten days on this dietary program. That's how long it takes for sufficiently large amounts of the beneficial fatty acids GLA and EPA to get into your inflammatory cells. I've done a number of studies on this subject, and, in asthmatics, it took just seven to ten days of supplementation with the right amounts and ratios of these fatty acids to see significant effects on the inflammatory messengers that cause the signs and symptoms of asthma.

If the scientific community knows that high levels of AA in foods are dangerous, why isn't this information out there already?

There's no conspiracy at work here, just a disconnect between the researchers who develop the science and the physicians who disseminate it among sick people. Scientists refer to this as "the research gap." By some estimates, it can take up to ten years for cutting-edge science to filter down to the people who need it the most!

In this case, the biochemists or molecular biologists who are doing the work on AA aren't focused on how their discoveries can best be used in a clinical setting. It's not that they aren't concentrating on "application"—of course they're thinking about helping people—but their focus tends to be more on understanding the mechanisms that lead to inflammatory diseases, and on developing medications like the terrific anti-inflammatory medications in your medicine cabinet right now. There has not yet been a real scientific focus on a dietary solution.

Your doctor hasn't been holding out on you either. Until now, a physician simply didn't have enough information to recommend a dietary program to help reduce inflammation safely and scientifically. The science is the major difference between my dietary program and other diets. No other program is backed by six clinical trials, or can point to results published in six peer-reviewed scientific journals. As this scientific information becomes widely disseminated, I believe the principles of the Chilton Program will become commonplace.

One of my principal intentions in writing this book is to help close that research gap, by bringing an all-natural, inflammation-reducing dietary program directly to doctors and their patients.

Will doing the Chilton Program disarm my inflammation system altogether, making it difficult for me to fight real infections?

The Chilton Program markedly reduces AA consumption, but does not eliminate it entirely. All of our clinical trials to date show that following the principles of the Chilton Program reduces but does not completely eliminate the production of inflammatory messengers. Your body should still be able to produce ample inflammatory messengers in order to fight infection.

How can I talk to my doctor about the Chilton Program?

I hope that you will talk to your doctor before beginning the Chilton Program. To make that process a little easier for you, I've included a "Letter to Your Doctor" starting on page 256 of this book, which summarizes the development of the science behind this dietary program.

In my experience, physicians have been very pleased to have a dietary program that they can recommend to help their patients with inflammatory disease, as long as there is rigorous science behind it. Although anti-inflammatory medications have been a godsend to sufferers, they don't necessarily go the whole distance, or work for everyone. Doctors, like their patients, tend to embrace anything that can help, especially when it comes backed by strong science.

Will eating according to the Chilton Program interfere with the way my medications work?

Absolutely not. It will probably give your medication an assist, but under no circumstances will eating according to the rules of the Chilton Program have any negative effect on the functionality of your medication.

Will the Chilton Program replace my medications?

I take the most conservative (and, in my opinion, ethical) approach to this question, so the answer is absolutely not. This is truly "complementary" medicine, by which I mean that this dietary program is designed to work synergistically *with* your medication, not as an alternative to it.

Have some people been able to reduce or eliminate their medications by following the rules of the Chilton Program? Yes. Some people, *working in close partnership with their physicians,* have been able to reduce the dosages of their maintenance medicines and the number of times they've had to turn to their rescue drugs. I will be as overjoyed as you are if correcting the balance of fatty acids in your diet makes you less dependent on medication—but I must insist that your doctor make any and all decisions about your medication protocols.

Does the program work differently for men and women?

There's no data in the scientific literature to suggest that men and women take up or process essential fatty acids differently. It is safe to assume that the Chilton Program should work equally well for men and women.

I'm petite, but my friend is not; can we both take the same supplement dose?

Yes. The reasons why are complicated, but clinical trials to date indicate that the doses I've provided are appropriate for adults of all sizes.

Will the Chilton Program stop an inflammatory disease flare-up?

The Chilton Program is a dietary maintenance system, not a rescue solution, which means that it is most effective in the *prevention* of flare-ups.

In almost all inflammatory diseases, there are "quiet" periods, characterized by minimal symptoms, and flare-ups, painful and periodic attacks. (If your disease is very severe, the flare-ups may occur so often as to appear constant.) Once the flare has begun, the proverbial horse is out of the barn, and no maintenance drug or dietary solution is going to help. This is why rescue drugs, like Albuterol for asthma sufferers, are so important.

But 70 percent of the asthma medications prescribed are maintenance medications, designed to *prevent* flares, just as the Chilton Program does. I would venture to say that this percentage is even higher in other inflammatory diseases. Flares are not only painful, but they cause lasting damage, so we have a great deal to gain from stopping them before they begin.

How will I know it's working?

You'll feel better. Based on our research, inflammatory messengers begin to fall within seven to ten days. Within that time, you should begin to see improvement in the symptoms of your inflammatory disease.

If that doesn't satisfy you, I have helped design two tests to measure your progress. One measures the incorporation of the fatty acids found in the Chilton Program into your bloodstream and the balance of those fatty acids. The other measures the levels of key inflammatory messengers (leukotrienes, in particular) produced by your body. Each of these tests can give you both a qualitative and quantitative indication of your improvement if you take them before you begin the Chilton Program, and then again after you've been doing the program for a little while. You and your doctor may want to do the test a few times in order to monitor your improvement.

For more information on these tests, go to www.biotechnicslab.com or www.inflammationnation.com, or write Biotechnics Lab, 310 Millstone Drive, Hillsborough, NC 27278.

Is the Chilton Program safe for my children?

There's certainly nothing harmful about the dietary portion of the program for children, and doing that part alone should be enough to see results.

We have done clinical trials in children using the rules of the Chilton Program, including GLA and EPA supplementation in children as young as age eleven. These trials, called pharmacokinetic trials, analyze how fast drugs are absorbed, distributed, and eliminated. Our trials revealed that children between eleven and eighteen years of age should ingest about 40 percent of the amount of GLA and EPA recommended for their adult counterparts in order to achieve the same blood levels of these fatty acids.

Taking this into consideration, I do believe that the entire program is safe for kids eleven to eighteen. But I absolutely don't think that parents should start their children on *any* program, especially one involving supplementation, without first consulting with their pediatrician. So while I do believe that the program is safe for children, I'd ask you to consult with a doctor, one who knows your kids, before beginning it with them.

Does having one inflammatory disease put me at higher risk for others?

Yes. As we saw in chapter 3, it's not unusual for a person living with one inflammatory disease to be much at higher risk for others.

For instance, people with eczema are at higher risk for asthma and allergies.

There's a commonsense reason for this. Inflammatory disease happens because the body is producing too many inflammatory messengers, bringing the overall level of inflammation in your body too high. That overproduction is causing the inflammatory disease you already have, and it can very well cause another one, too. The Chilton Program lowers the overall levels of inflammatory messengers, so it can not only help to address the inflammatory disease you already have, but also help to prevent the onset of others—or the onset of inflammatory disease altogether, if you've been lucky enough to dodge the bullet thus far.

I make sure to purchase "organic" salmon. Is it lower in AA?

Not necessarily. Organic salmon is farmed, and although the regulations are stricter for organic fish farmers than for ordinary aquaculture, those regulations may not address the inflammation issue. Organic salmon live in less crowded pens, they're fed a better quality of fish meal, and they aren't fed a synthetic pigment to make their flesh pink. But as far as I know, there is no research to suggest that organic salmon are lower in preformed AA than other farm-raised salmon.

There is no research to suggest that organic salmon is less contaminated with PCBs and dioxin, either. This isn't to say that it isn't true, just that it hasn't, to my knowledge, been conclusively proven. There's also a question about what "organic" means in this context. The National Organics Program of the USDA does not yet have standards that apply to seafood, which is why you don't see the USDA's organic seal stuck in the ice next to the fish. In fact, the only regulatory agencies are in Europe.

What happens if I cheat?

It depends on what you mean by cheating. If you're asking what happens if you eat a piece of birthday cake (high on the Glycemic Index, and therefore a violation of the third strategy) once in a while, the answer is "not much." If you eat a piece of cake every day, that's a different story.

The same thing is true for the fatty-acid balance. If you forget your GLA supplement one day, will your inflammation return at pre-program levels? No. Your inflammatory messengers will return to pre-program levels fairly rapidly, though, if you fail to maintain the correct balance of fatty acids in your diet. In a recent study, my laboratory demonstrated that it took about two weeks of being "off" those critical fatty acids for the inflammatory messengers that cause asthma to return to their pre-program levels.

The short answer is, yes, you can cheat. That said, I would advise you to stick to the program as closely as possible. With every day that you're on the healthy balance of fatty acids in the Chilton Program, your cells and tissues are replacing inappropriate fatty acids from your Western diet. Likewise, the longer you replace the fatty acids in the Chilton Program with the fatty acids in your Western diet, the longer it will take to correct that imbalance.

Is there a stress component to inflammatory disease?

There is a great deal of anecdotal evidence to suggest that stress and other psychological factors play a role in inflammatory disease and in the timing and severity of inflammatory disease flares. However, there's no convincing scientific evidence to confirm this. This is why the Chilton Program is restricted to diet, and does not extend to stress-management techniques like doing meditation or yoga, or enjoying a beer by the pool. If you find that these strategies, or any others, help you to manage your disease, then I wholeheartedly encourage you to pursue them. They will certainly not hurt you, and may help—if not your inflammatory disease, then in other areas of your life.

What about foods I've heard are anti-inflammatory, like onions?

You may have heard that some foods have anti-inflammatory properties, including members of the allium family (onions, garlic, leeks, and shallots), ginger, honey, pineapple, papaya, turmeric, and apples.

Again, the anecdotal evidence for the anti-inflammatory properties of these foods is much stronger than the scientific evidence, so I don't specifically recommend that you eat them as part of the Chilton Program. That said, these foods make delicious and healthful additions to any diet, so I certainly won't dissuade you from adding them to yours.

Do I have to do the diet? Are there any shortcuts?

The answer is "not really." The best way to do this program is to change the way you eat, for a number of reasons:

◆ First of all, I believe that eating according to the Chilton Program, with its focus on whole foods, nutrient-dense carbohydrates, and lean proteins with low concentrations of AA and beneficial fatty acids, is a healthful way to eat. I believe it is a much healthier diet, for instance, than the typical one that most Americans follow.

◆ There's no shortcut for monitoring your AA intake. If you want to see a reduction in inflammation, you must keep your daily Inflammatory Index value within the parameters of the diet you're following (below 150 for prevention, and 100 for solution).

◆ You *must* restrict your carbohydrate intake to foods with low-to-moderate values on the Glycemic Index.

So I believe that the best way to do this program is to eat utilizing the strategies of the program as they appear in this book.

That said, the Chilton Program isn't something that you'll be doing for two weeks; it's a way of eating that I hope you'll integrate fully into your daily life. I understand that sometimes life interferes with the best-laid plans. You may not be able to eat four Category 1 fish every week; you may have other dietary restrictions that make this impossible for you, or you may simply not like fish. If this is the case, rest assured: as long as you are prepared to monitor your carbohydrate intake using the Glycemic Index, and to monitor your AA intake using the Inflammatory Index, you can make up the amount of EPA you need to follow the rules of the Chilton Program using supplements. For more information on the best sources of fatty-acid dietary supplements, please go to www.inflammation nation.com.

I've heard about Airozin and Solaira. What is it and do I have to take it? How can it help me?

Over the past five years, a company that I founded, called Pilot Therapeutics, has been developing a medical food called Airozin. Airozin is the subject of several patents. This medical food will provide specially formulated, highly enriched fatty acids—specifically, GLA and EPA, in the amounts and ratios that have been clinically proven to reduce the inflammatory messengers known to cause flares in inflammatory disease. There may be some benefit to taking GLA and EPA in the form of a medical food like Airozin. In fact, approximately twice as much GLA is delivered to inflammatory cells when GLA is provided as part of the Airozin emulsion as it is when taken in a gel capsule. So you need to take less of these fatty acids in order to reduce inflammatory messengers.

Airozin is a creamy, orange-flavored liquid emulsion packed in once-a-day, foil packets. Two separate formulas are being developed, one for individuals age six to eleven and one for those twelve and older. Like the Chilton Program, Airozin is not a rescue medication; it should be viewed as a long-term management solution for inflammatory diseases. It is not intended to replace medications.

Unlike most natural-food companies, we have invested the time and money with clinical trials necessary to determine that Airozin is worthy of human consumption—and safe. Several peer-reviewed scientific articles document the discovery of Airozin and verify that it is safe and effective. We have now developed a dietary supplement gel capsule system, called Solaira, that delivers the precise concentrations and ratios of GLA and EPA.

Again, I would like to emphasize this important point: if you are already taking GLA or EPA as a supplement, or if you are consuming large amounts of these fatty acids as part of your diet, DO NOT take additional GLA or EPA in the form of Airozin or Solaira.

For more information on Airozin and Solaira, please go to www.solaira.info or www.inflammationnation.com.

I did not write this book to sell the products that I have developed; you'll do just as well altering your diet and using GLA and EPA supplements from the health-food store. I simply offer them here as an alternative if the Chilton Program, for whatever reason, is difficult for you to follow. If you do take the medical food route, please remember, as I have said many times, that even the best fatty-acid products are not effective unless dietary AA and carbohydrate levels are monitored.

Will the Chilton Program help everyone?

Nothing helps everyone. The Chilton Program can help many people, but not everyone. Whether or not the Chilton Program—or any dietary intervention—can help you is largely based on your genetic makeup. One of the newest disciplines in medicine is called nutragenomics, the combination of how our diets and our genes affect our health. Some people are "diet responders." If you're a diet responder to sodium, then your blood pressure will go down if you cut down the amount of salt in your diet. If you're a cholesterol diet responder, then your risk factors for heart disease will look much better after you've reduced the amount of saturated fat in your diet. And if you're an AA diet responder, then you will produce fewer inflammatory messengers if you follow the rules of the Chilton Program.

Not everyone, however, is a diet responder—in the same way that not everyone responds to the inflammation-quieting medications on the market. However, I do believe that the Chilton Program will have a wide application. I believe that we as humans were genetically designed to eat according to the rules of this dietary program. Consequently, I believe my program will have broader applications than many medications, and may offer a beacon of hope to some of those people for whom medication does not work.

PART 3

Tools for Healthy Living

Chapter Ten
What's Your IQ?

The results of this informal quiz, which takes the form of three sets of questions, will deliver your IQ—and by IQ, I don't mean your Intelligence Quotient, but instead your *Inflammatory Quotient*.

Why Take This Test?

There are two reasons to take this test.

The first is to discover whether or not you (or a loved one) has an inflammatory disease. You'd be surprised at how few people know the underlying cause behind the illnesses that affect them. If I'm meeting someone and I say that I conduct research on inflammatory diseases, their eyes glaze over. Most of the time, they don't even bother to ask me what that means. But if I say I study the mechanism behind allergies, asthma, and arthritis, the reaction is radically different. Suddenly, people are popping out of the woodwork with a story to tell, a question to ask, a theory to put forth.

It is true that for some of you, the very concept of an "inflammatory quiz" is redundant: inflammatory disease is something you live with every day. I'd recommend that you read this chapter anyway, for one reason: it may enable you to help someone you care about, someone who has not yet been hit by the tidal wave.

There's another reason to take this quiz, and that reason is *risk*. You may unwittingly be at risk for inflammatory disease—and you may unwittingly be engaging in behaviors that put you directly in the line of fire. If you already have inflammatory disease, you may be at risk of contracting another, if you're doing things that increase your overall level of inflammation.

Although we're all feeding from the same poisoned trough, not everyone will contract an inflammatory disease. Some of us are genetically predisposed to it, and some of our behaviors may exacerbate that risk. You cannot change many of the factors that contribute to inflammatory disease. Don't you want to control the ones you can?

This extremely informal assessment of your level of overall inflammation will also guide you to which level of the Chilton Program (Prevention or Solution) is most appropriate for you.

The Chilton IQ Quiz

Part One Answer the following questions by checking off each one that applies.

Have you been diagnosed with

_____ asthma?

_____ seasonal allergies or hay fever?

_____ eczema?

_____ atopic (allergic) dermatitis?

_____ contact dermatitis?

_____ rheumatoid arthritis?

_____ lupus?

_____ scleroderma?

_____ inflammatory bowel disease (IBD)?

_____ gout?

_____ Crohn's disease?

_____ ulcerative colitis?

_____ sprue?

_____ psoriasis?

_____ allergies to pet dander, dust, or dust mites?

_____ a disease that causes you to routinely take drugs called corticosteroids, such as prednisone?

If you checked off any of the conditions in this section, you have an inflammatory disease. You may benefit from further tests such as the ones found at the end of this chapter.

Since you already have an inflammatory disease, you need active intervention, and I believe you will benefit from following the Chilton Solution Program found in this book (meal plans for this program begin on page 206).

If you checked off none of the conditions above, please continue with part two of the quiz.

Part Two Answer the following questions by checking off each one that applies.

Do you have

_____ hardening of the arteries (atherosclerosis)?

_____ chronic kidney failure?

_____ chronic hepatitis?

_____ chronic thyroid disease?

_____ chronic pancreatitis?

_____ Alzheimer's disease?

_____ osteoarthritis?

_____ chronic bronchitis or chronic obstructive

pulmonary disease (COPD) including emphysema?

_____ food allergies?

_____ high levels of C-reactive protein (CRP)?

_____ parents or siblings who have been diagnosed with one of the diseases listed in part one of the quiz?

Have you had

_____ a heart attack?   _____ a stroke?

If you checked off any of the conditions in this section, you have a significant risk of inflammatory disease. You may benefit from further tests such as the ones found at the end of this chapter. Since your risk is significant, I believe you will benefit from following the Chilton Solution Program found in this book (again, meal plans for this program begin on page 206).

If you checked off none of the conditions above, please continue with part three of the quiz.

Part Three Answer the following questions by checking off each one that applies.

Do you

_____ have chronic high blood pressure that is difficult to control?

_____ have cancer of the colon, stomach, lung, or breast?

_____ have parents or siblings who could answer yes to any of the questions in part two of the quiz?

_____ take drugs to control your cholesterol or triglycerides?

_____ smoke regularly and have a chronic cough?

_____ eat eggs more than three times a week?

_____ eat salmon more than three times a week? Do you know if it's farmed or wild?

_____ have recurring gum problems or gum disease?

_____ you have an injured joint? Have you ever had surgery on a joint?

_____ Is your body mass index (BMI) more than 30? (Please see page 159 for more information on how to calculate your BMI.)

If you checked off any of the conditions in this section, you have a *moderate* risk of inflammatory disease. You may benefit from further tests such as the ones found at the end of this chapter. Since your risk is moderate, I believe you should consider following the Chilton Prevention Program found in this book (meal plans for this program begin on page 177).

If you checked off none of the conditions in this chapter, congratulations. It sounds as if you're inflammation free!

Further Testing

If your quiz came back with some positive answers, you may benefit from further testing to determine with more specificity the level of inflammation in your blood.

C-Reactive Protein (CRP)

One of the only existing tests for inflammation is a test called high-sensitivity C-reactive protein, otherwise known as CRP. This protein is released into the bloodstream whenever there is serious inflammation in the body; it's designed to help the body defend itself. When the inflammation is chronic and persistent, levels of CRP will appear high. This test is being used more and more to determine a patient's level of risk for heart disease. One study showed that people with high CRP were four to seven times more likely to develop heart disease than people with normal levels. And in another large study, high CRP was a better predictor of heart attack than LDL, or "bad" cholesterol. It also appears that people with high levels of CRP are more likely to have a second heart attack.

Is CRP a good indicator of other inflammatory diseases? Currently, there is not enough scientific data to say definitively. We do know that it has been used with some initial success for assessing inflammation in patients with rheumatoid arthritis.

Two New Tests

I have worked closely with Biotechnics Lab to develop two tests that, together and apart, will help to ascertain your inflammatory potential and the level of inflammatory messengers in your body.

The first test is a blood test that must be done in coordination with your physician. It measures the amounts of certain polyunsaturated fatty acids in the blood. You'll recognize them: AA (arachidonic acid), EPA (eicosapentanoic acid), DHA (docasahexanoic acid), GLA (gamma-linolenic acid), and DGLA (dihomogammalinolenic acid).

The second test, which can be done by you in your own home, determines the levels of leukotrienes made by your body by looking at these inflammatory messengers and their metabolites (the substances produced by their interaction with other chemicals) in your urine.

Used together, these tests are a good way to determine your inflammatory potential, and whether or not the Chilton Program is working: with the first test, you'll be able to determine the critical fatty-acid ratios in your blood and whether or not the fatty-acid ratios in your blood have changed as a result of your new eating patterns; with the second test, you'll be able to tell whether or not you're producing fewer of the inflammatory messengers that lead to the signs and symptoms of inflammatory disease.

For more information on these tests, go to www.inflammationnation .com or www.biotechnicslab.com, or write Biotechnics Lab, 310 Millstone Drive, Hillsborough, NC 27278.

Congratulations. You have taken a major step toward better health and a rebalanced immune system simply by picking up this book and committing yourself to changing the way you eat.

If you're still reading, I'm going to assume that you're convinced—convinced that an incorrectly balanced diet is playing a major role behind this inflammatory epidemic and your own inflammatory disease or risk of disease, and convinced that the Chilton Program can help you to bring your diet back into balance.

An Eating Plan That You Can Live With

I've looked at the other anti-inflammatory diets out there, but I wasn't convinced by the science.

But let's say, for argument's sake, that those diets represent the most cutting-edge research out there. *I still don't think they'd make you better.* Why? Because I think you'd be sneaking out to get some real, filling, good-tasting food before the first week was up. You'd have to be very, very sick to stick with these rigid, punishing diets. And as far as I'm concerned, a diet that doesn't work in the real world is a diet that doesn't work. As every self-help book will tell you, in order to make real and lasting changes in your life, you'll need to find a way to incorporate them into your lifestyle fully.

If you've read those other books, tried those diets, and despaired, I have a piece of good news to deliver: this time will be different. I'll tell you now what I told Linda Easter, the nutritionist who helped to put the meal plans and recipes together: "I'm not putting people on a diet I won't do myself." I'm not the healthiest eater in the world, and I don't think you have to be, either.

Yes, I will ask you to avoid certain foods, but they're easily substituted for. Indeed, I believe most dieters have been waiting a long time to have someone tell them that it's okay to swap out certain kinds of salmon for a lean steak!

On the Chilton Program, you won't go hungry, and you won't have to eat twigs. Food is central to the quality of our lives, and hunger is possibly our most powerful drive. It's unrealistic to think that something this important can be marginalized, or that you can spend the rest of your life denying yourself. I can assure you that the hunter-gatherers didn't keep food journals, or obsess over whether their fatty-acid balance was healthy—they ate what was available and what they were used to eating. Ultimately, the point of the Chilton Program is to educate you so that you can make the healthiest choices for your situation.

For some of you, the easiest way to do that may be to follow a very specific roadmap until you get your bearings. That's why we've included four weeks of meal plans for both the Prevention and Solution Diets in this book. If you're not the kind of person who likes to ask directions, I'd encourage you to think of these meal plans as guidelines, and to rely more heavily on the indexes.

The meal plans themselves aren't set in stone; there is some flexibility built in. For instance, you should always feel free to substitute one food with another, as long as it has roughly the same Inflammatory Index rating. And if strawberries come into season just as you start this program, by all means, substitute them for an apple. Mix and match lunches and dinners, as long as you keep your Inflammatory Index value for the day under the recommended amount. Some additional guidelines:

Menu Preparation

- ◆ Fruit may be fresh, canned, or frozen as long as it is unsweetened.
- ◆ Vegetables may be fresh or frozen. Canned vegetables should be used only when nothing else is available; they are inferior both in taste and nutritional value to fresh and frozen alternatives.

- ◆ All margarine used is 70 percent vegetable oil spread containing no trans fats.
- ◆ Fats (oil, margarine, salad dressings, and mayonnaise) may be used only when indicated. If no fat is listed, nonstick cooking spray or butter-flavored granules may be used.
- ◆ Menus provide suggested distribution of foods across three meals and one snack; however, you can eat the foods in whatever combination you desire.
- ◆ Low-fat cheeses are 2 percent milk cheeses, with approximately 2 grams of fat per ounce.
- ◆ All juices are unsweetened or artificially sweetened.
- ◆ Unsweetened or artificially sweetened beverages, including coffee, tea, water, and diet sodas, may be used as desired.
- ◆ The following flavorings, seasonings, and spices may be used as desired: garlic; herbs (like basil, oregano, thyme); spices (like salt, pepper, cinnamon, nutmeg); lemon juice for seasoning; vinegars; sugar substitutes.

I'd encourage you to think of this as an opportunity. These meal plans take into account an astonishing range of nutritional parameters. Not only are the foods included low on the Inflammatory Index, but they also are low in saturated fat and include the polyunsaturated fats that our bodies need to function properly.

National and international guidelines for prevention of heart disease recommend that saturated fat stay below 10 percent of calories, polyunsaturated above 7 percent, monounsaturated above 10 percent, dietary cholesterol below 300 milligrams a day, and that daily fiber be increased to more than 25 grams a day. When you eat the Chilton way, you will improve on those guidelines. On the Chilton Solution Diet, your average daily (AD) amount of saturated fats is 8.8 percent of calories, the polyunsaturated fat is 9.1 percent of calories, monosaturated fat is 15.4 percent of caloric intake, and your AD cholesterol intake is at 224 milligrams. Your daily fiber intake is 30.1 grams. On the Prevention Diet, the AD amount of saturated fat is 8.7 percent of calories, polyunsaturated fat makes up 9.7 percent of calories, and monosaturated fat is 16.8 percent of calories. Your dietary cholesterol is 251 milligrams, and your daily fiber intake is 30.1 grams. The meal plans in this book are designed not only to be anti-inflammatory, but to present you with a more healthful way to eat. Enjoy it—and the way you feel as a result!

Talk to Your Doctor

The first thing you should do before beginning the Chilton Program is have a conversation with your doctor.

Because maintenance and the prevention of flares is such an enormous part of treating inflammatory disease, and because the medications for severe inflammatory disease have the potential to be toxic, physicians who treat inflammatory disease tend to be open to discussing complementary diet and supplementation programs with their patients as long as the proposed programs are backed by real science, as this one is.

I have included a "Letter to Your Doctor" from me (starting on page 256), which summarizes the program and what I believe it can do for inflammatory disease sufferers. There are also two tests, explained on page 145, that will enable your doctor to measure your progress. Don't skip this step: you need your doctor's okay to go forward, and you need his or her reassurance that the supplements I suggest won't interfere or react badly with other medications that you're taking.

Pick Your Supplements Carefully

Supplementation is a significant part of the Chilton Program.

Americans are considerably more used to the idea of supplementing their diets than they once were. A study published in the *American Journal of Preventative Medicine* found that half of all Americans take a vitamin or mineral supplement, and the researchers noted that much of that supplementation was associated with various medical conditions.

In this book, I recommend that you take a supplement of gamma-linoleic acid (GLA). Look for a GLA supplement that comes from borage seed oil. In certain circumstances I also recommend that you take a supplement of eicosapentanoic acid (EPA).

You should take an EPA supplement if

- ◆ you are on the Chilton Prevention Diet, and are not able to eat at least three meals per week of Category 1 or 2 fish. (See the Chilton Fish Ranking for a list of fish in these categories.)
- ◆ you are on the Chilton Solution Diet, and are not able to eat at least four meals a week of Category 1 or 2 fish. (See the Chilton Fish Ranking for a list of fish in these categories.)

For specific dosage information, please see chapter 16.

If you are unable to eat the recommended amount of fish, but you can eat some fish, I recommend that you adjust the amount of supplement you take accordingly. This doesn't need to be a complicated calculation. For instance, if you eat two Category 2 fish meals this week (which is a little more than half the recommended dosage for the Chilton Prevention Diet), you need to take only half the recommended supplement dose. In this case, as you'll see in chapter 16, that means taking just one capsule a day of an EPA supplement.

Please note: just because these supplement products are "natural" doesn't mean they're harmless. In fact, one of the supplements I recommend for this program, GLA, has potentially dangerous side effects if it is taken *without* EPA, another fatty acid that acts as a blocker for that side effect. **DO NOT take the recommended doses of GLA without having EPA—either through the fish that you're eating, or by supplementation—in your diet. You would be better off not taking anything than taking the wrong thing.**

I'd also encourage you to stick to my dosage recommendations. At too low a dose, these products won't do much; at too high a dose, they can have adverse effects. If you're unable to follow the Chilton Program, a gel capsule system called Solaira has been developed that delivers the precise dosage and ratios of GLA and EPA (see chapter 9).

The Food and Drug Administration (FDA) tests medications extensively before it approves their use; no such rigorous tests are required to market and sell supplements. Since they aren't regulated, there can be some inconsistency in the way the oils are extracted, the base they're in, and their strength. Personally, there are several things that I look at before using a supplier.

For example, does the company

- accept raw materials from Good Manufacturing Practice (GMP)–approved facilities only?
- conduct supplier audits and inspect their suppliers' facilities?
- insist that its suppliers register with the FDA in compliance with the new bioterrorism legislation, and, in the case of plant oils, are they able to show traceability back to the farmer who produced the product?
- process its EPA products to pharmaceutical-quality standards, using molecular or steam distillation?
- minimally process its GLA products and not hexane-extract them?
- have national distribution?
- dedicate itself to helping educate consumers on essential fatty acids?

For more information on these criteria, see www.inflammation nation.com.

Get Your Kitchen Ready

Clean out your cupboards. Sticking to foods that rank low to moderate on the Glycemic Index is very important on the Chilton Program, so if you're someone for whom willpower is a problem, I'd recommend that you eliminate potentially tempting items from your cupboards before you even begin the program.

While you're at it, replace all the unhealthy corn and "vegetable" oils with canola and olive oil, and get rid of all the white pasta, rice, and white flour.

Check the sugar content! You'd be surprised how much sugar lurks in commercial tomato and barbeque sauces, ketchup, and fruit-based drinks. Check labels for ingredients such as glucose, fructose, sucrose, corn syrup, high fructose corn syrup, molasses, honey, dextrose, sorghum, lactose, maltose, or concentrated grape juice. If you see these ingredients, there's sugar hiding in there.

Drink in moderation. Alcohol is low in carbohydrates, but your body processes it in a way that's similar to the way it handles glucose, and that can spell trouble for your insulin levels. I don't have a problem if you drink a couple of glasses of wine throughout the week, but heavy drinking in one sitting is out.

What about caffeine? There's no reason not to continue enjoying coffee or tea if a cup or two a day is part of your ordinary regimen. But remember, sugar is a no-no.

Buy a fish cookbook. Since you're going to be eating a great deal more fish when you do the Chilton Program, it might be worth investing in a good book of fish cookery. We've provided you with recipes in this book to get you started, but if you've never prepared fish before, you may want more details about the basics—and, as delicious as the recipes we've provided are, you will probably want to broaden your horizons eventually.

Chapter Twelve
Losing Weight on the Chilton Program

There's an old Doonesbury cartoon that I love. It dates from the height of the Jane Fonda exercise craze, and in it, Jane cries: "Male diet doctors hid the truth from me: eat less and exercise!"

The truth is a little more complicated than that cartoon panel, but not much. I wish there was a magic bullet I could give you to help you to lose weight, something you haven't heard before. There isn't. The best I can do is present this information in a way that makes sense to me, in the hopes that it will make sense to you.

Our eating habits have fallen out of balance, with the result that we're no longer eating the way we were designed to eat. The rise in processed and "fast" foods has given way to highly caloric, nutrient-poor foods, often in the form of refined carbohydrates and sugars as well as unbalanced fatty acids. This trend, in my opinion, has led to an epidemic rise in diseases related not just to obesity, but to inflammation as well. Fighting obesity is part of fighting inflammatory disorders. As you have seen in this book, it is only part of that solution. But to fight both, we must change the way we eat.

The Input/Output Equation

It may not be as simple as "eat less and exercise," but the first and most important part of losing weight is to understand the following: the food you put into your body is either burned or stored.

The measure for determining how much energy a food contains is called a kilocalorie, com-

> The food you put into your body is either burned or stored.

monly referred to as a calorie. Every packaged food sold in the United States is required to contain caloric information. You burn a certain number of calories simply by existing; think of your body as a car on idle. And like that car, the more you move—and the faster you go—the more fuel, in the form of calories, you burn.

More Than Calories Alone

If the calories you put into your body are either burned or stored, then is it okay to eat doughnuts until you hit your personal calorie limit for the day? You can probably guess the answer to that one.

The truth is that weight loss is a little more complicated than calories in and calories out.

Here's why. A glazed, raspberry-filled doughnut (my favorite) contains 350 calories. Now, I personally need 2,686 calories per day to maintain my current body weight. (I'll show you how to figure out how many calories you need in a moment.) So that means I can eat about seven of those delicious raspberry-filled confections, and I'd still be eating few enough calories to lose weight. Right?

Not so fast. As facetious as my doughnut example may seem, it's actually a very extreme representation of the typical American diet, a diet that I believe bears much responsibility for the epidemic of obesity in this country—as it does for the epidemic of inflammatory disease. Let's use this extreme doughnut example to look at the problem of the way Americans think about food.

First of all, the foods we eat are calorie-rich, but they're not filling. I'm going to scarf a 350-calorie doughnut down in three bites. It won't fill my belly, or make the slightest dent in my hunger. In fact, once my blood sugar has spiked and crashed again, I'm likely to find myself even hungrier than I was *before* I had the doughnut. It's the very definition of a quick fix.

And yet, that doughnut represents a significant portion of the calories I can eat for the day, and with very few nutrients to show for it. This is what people mean when they call food items like doughnuts "empty calories." Donuts are very expensive from a calorie standpoint, but without much return: they're not good for you, and they don't fill you up. The exact opposite is true for fiber-rich, filling, and nutritious vegetables. For the same 350 calories as that doughnut, I can eat satisfying portions, which will leave me full, with tons of health-giving vitamins, minerals, and phytonutrients, the potent antioxidants in fruit and vegetable pigments, thrown into the bargain.

Now, I'm not suggesting that you sit down to an endless bag of carrots for breakfast, lunch, and dinner, but you can see how the calories add up when a sugary snack like a doughnut gobbles up such a significant portion of my daily calorie allotment without providing significant nutritional benefit, or without even filling me up! You can easily recognize how we get into trouble. I'm human, and if I'm hungry, I'm going to eat until I get full. If my food choices are concentrated on calorie-rich, nutrient-poor, fundamentally unsatisfying foods like cookies and doughnuts, I'm going to end up taking in a lot more calories than my body really needs—which will eventually manifest in a roll of fat around my waist.

Calorie density isn't the only reason we're facing an upswing in obesity-related disease. In the United States, the food we eat tends to be highly processed, and we're only just discovering how dangerous some of these processing methods are. For instance, there has been much in the news recently about trans-fatty acids. These are fats that have been chemically altered to make them more stable (so they can sit on a supermarket shelf for a long time) and to give the products in which they're found a better texture, or "mouth-feel." They're used in a variety of household staples, including packaged bakery items, cookies, crackers, and peanut butter.

These fatty acids increase LDL, or "bad" cholesterol concentrations, and since LDL is unquestionably connected to risk of heart disease, we should reduce our intake of these cholesterol-raising fatty acids. The USDA has mandated that foods containing trans-fatty acids be labeled, but that won't happen until 2006. In the meantime, margarine, shortening, or partially hydrogenated soybean oil can contain high concentrations of these fats. When they do, they should be avoided.

You'll find that not all margarines are created equal, and some contain small quantities of, or no, trans-fatty acids and thus have negligible effects on the cholesterol levels.

Like the disproportionate distribution of fatty acids in our diets, this is the result of industrialization: trans fats are necessary because a food made with a more natural fat like butter would be rancid by the time it left the factory, never mind the time it took to ship that product to a supermarket, where it sits on a shelf until you put it in your cart and take it home. But industrialization shouldn't necessarily mean that we commit to eating in a way we're not designed to eat.

For years, epidemiologists have struggled with the "French Paradox." Although the French diet is filled with fatty pâtés and foie gras and steak and butter, the French are not only much thinner, but they have much lower incidence of heart disease than Americans do. A number of theories have been put forth to explain this. One credits the heart-healthy benefits of the red wine that the French drink, but most cardiologists think there has to be more to it than wine. Another theory is that the French have better portion control than Americans do; while that's true, I believe it's only part of the whole picture.

I think one of the secrets behind the French Paradox is this: the French eat more whole foods, and foods that contain the proper polyunsaturated fatty-acid balance. The French eat more fish than Americans do. Animals raised in France have leaner meat than ours do, and the French don't eat fast food, or drink soda in the amounts that we do, or snack on chips and cookies. As a result, they eat much less sugar, many fewer refined carbohydrates, fewer trans fats—and a much healthier balance of the fatty acids that contribute both to inflammation and obesity.

And of course, as I mentioned above, the French have better portion control! The whole foods they eat are *more filling*—so they need to eat less of it to feel full. You'll find the same thing to be true with the foods you're eating on the Chilton Program: whole foods fill you up, so you need to eat less to feel satisfied.

The Carbohydrate Connection

I believe it's in Americans' dependence on (one might even say addiction to) "foods of affluence" like doughnuts that the connection between the epidemics in inflammation and obesity collide. Specifically, the amount and the quality of the carbohydrates in the typical American diet are out of control.

It's here that the obesity and inflammatory epidemics overlap, as shown in the figure below.

> The amount and the *quality* of the carbohydrates in the typical American diet are out of control.

There are two separate issues: both the amount and the *quality* of the carbohydrates we eat are out of whack. Vegetables have carbohydrates, you'll no doubt point out. But I'm pretty sure that 64 percent of Americans aren't overweight or obese because they've been overdoing the five-veggies-a-day rule.

It's the quality of the carbohydrates we're eating that's doing us in. It's the highly refined starches and sugars we're consuming at an unprecedented rate: the soda, the beer, the candy, the chips, the French fries, the white bread—and, yes, the doughnuts—that have gotten us into trouble. Now anyone who knows me knows that I'm not constitutionally opposed to the occasional treat: a cookie over coffee with a friend, a piece of birth-

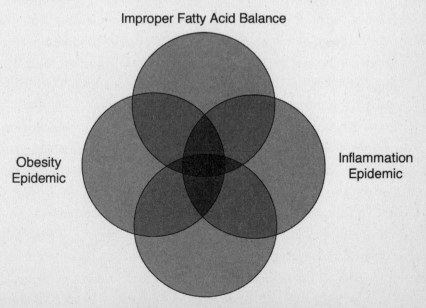

Relationships Among Fatty Acid and Carbohydrate
Balance and the Inflammation and Obesity Epidemics

Improper Fatty Acid Balance

Obesity
Epidemic

Inflammation
Epidemic

Improper Carbohydrate Balance

day cake, a cold beer at a Fourth of July barbeque. Unfortunately, most of us don't view these items as occasional treats, rather we use them as our most basic fuel; that's how we're eating ourselves sick.

Those processed sugars and carbohydrates are making us fat. But they're contributing to the inflammatory epidemic as well.

As you'll remember from chapter 3, high levels of glucose and insulin are linked to the production of inflammatory messengers from AA. Additionally, high levels of insulin activate the enzyme that generates AA in the human body. Insulin and the inflammatory messengers made from AA have a symbiotic, interregulatory relationship as well, and those messengers also appear to control how rapidly insulin removes glucose from the bloodstream. In chapter 3, we learned that obesity is a chronic inflammatory condition, and one intimately linked to the production of inflammatory messengers, which in turn triggers insulin resistance, syndrome X, and diabetes.

The take-home message is this: our "diets of affluence" have wreaked havoc with interconnected systems throughout our body.

How the Chilton Program Can Help

Our out-of-control carbohydrate and fatty-acid consumption has given rise to the epidemic in obesity and obesity-related disease, and there is a clear link between inflammatory disease and being overweight. Attacking these issues is a major way that the Chilton Program addresses both weight loss and controlling rampant inflammation.

The kinds of fatty acids we eat, and the ratios in which we eat them, are out of whack, leading to this epidemic in inflammatory disease. The types of carbohydrates we eat, and the quantities in which we eat them, are out of whack as well, and this disproportion is again strongly linked to the increase in inflammatory disease. We're not designed to eat fifty-six teaspoonfuls of sugar every day! As a result, strategies for bringing our carbohydrate consumption—the quality and the quantity—under control is one of the major focuses of the dietary program to come.

I don't really call the Chilton Program a low-carbohydrate, high-protein diet. That phrase presupposes that the typical American diet is a "normal" and "balanced" baseline—and I believe that nothing could be farther from the truth.

The foods you'll eat on my diet, and the proportions in which you'll eat them, are more in line with the way that I believe that our bodies were designed to eat. Please—don't think of this diet as low or high in any one particular macronutrient; think of it as pulling all elements of your diet back into balance. Yes, compared to the typical American diet, the Chilton Program surely is low-carb. It has to be. We've already seen the devastation wrought by changes in the kinds of food that we eat and the ways those foods are produced. And I believe we've paid the price, in those twin tidal waves of obesity and inflammatory diseases. We must now correct our course.

Are You Overweight?

The first question to answer is: Are you overweight?

Our national body image is unbelievably skewed. On the one hand, we're surrounded by idealized images of very thin people, in movies, on TV, in magazines. On the other, we're battling a nationwide crisis in obesity. According to the June 2004 issue of the *Journal of the American Medical Association*, 64 percent of the adults in this country are either overweight or obese.

Diagnosing the problem is always a good place to start. In fact, there is a relatively simple way to determine whether or not you're overweight—and how overweight you are, if that's the case. It's called the Body Mass Index. There's an equation to determine your own personal BMI, but a chart is quicker and easier: find the box where your height and current weight meet. The number at the top of the column is your BMI. To determine where your BMI falls on the healthy weight continuum (as determined by the National Institutes of Health), consult the table that follows.

Body Mass Index

Height in Inches	19	20	21	22	23	24	25	26	27	28	29	30	31	32	33	34	35
	Body Weight (pounds)																
58	91	96	100	105	110	115	119	124	129	134	138	143	148	153	158	162	167
59	94	99	104	109	114	119	124	128	133	138	143	148	153	158	163	168	173
60	97	102	107	112	118	123	128	133	138	143	148	153	158	163	168	174	179
61	100	106	111	116	122	127	132	137	143	148	153	158	164	169	174	180	185
62	104	109	115	120	126	131	136	142	147	153	158	164	169	175	180	186	191
63	107	113	118	124	130	135	141	146	152	158	163	169	175	180	186	191	197
64	110	116	122	128	134	140	145	151	157	163	169	174	180	186	192	197	204
65	114	120	126	132	138	144	150	156	162	168	174	180	186	192	198	204	210
66	118	124	130	136	142	148	155	161	167	173	179	186	192	198	204	210	216
67	121	127	134	140	146	153	159	166	172	178	185	191	198	204	211	217	223
68	125	131	138	144	151	158	164	171	177	184	190	197	203	210	216	223	230
69	128	135	142	149	155	162	169	176	182	189	196	203	209	216	223	230	236
70	132	139	146	153	160	167	174	181	188	195	202	209	216	222	229	236	243
71	136	143	150	157	165	172	179	186	193	200	208	215	222	229	236	243	250
72	140	147	154	162	169	177	184	191	199	206	213	221	228	235	242	250	258
73	144	151	159	166	174	182	189	197	204	212	219	227	235	242	250	257	265
74	148	155	163	171	179	186	194	202	210	218	225	233	241	249	256	264	272
75	152	160	168	176	184	192	200	208	216	224	232	240	248	256	264	272	279
76	156	164	172	180	189	197	205	213	221	230	238	246	254	263	271	279	287

<18.5	Underweight
18.5–24.9	Healthy Weight
25–29.9	Overweight
30+	Obese

NOT A PERFECT INSTRUMENT

The BMI is not a perfect tool, so you should use yours as a guideline, not a rule. First of all, your BMI may appear to be high if you're very muscular. And although it serves our purposes here, many physicians, especially cardiologists, have grown dissatisfied with the BMI, particularly when used as a potential indicator of heart disease. A better measurement, perhaps, is some combination of BMI and waist circumference, which may be a better indicator (people who get fat around their middle have a higher risk of heart disease than people who carry weight in their hips and thighs and rear end). To escape the heart disease high-risk zone, a man's waist measured around the navel should be less than forty inches; a woman's less than thirty-five.

If you're a healthy weight, congratulations! You're certainly in the minority. If you'd like to continue reading this chapter, you may discover some interesting information about how your weight—specifically excess fat—affects inflammatory disease.

> If you eat the way your body was designed to, your weight loss wiil be easier than it's ever been before.

If, like so many Americans, you are overweight, keep reading. All is not lost! In fact, when you're eating the way your body was designed to eat, you may discover that weight loss is easier than it ever has been before, because you're working with your body, not against it.

Determine Your Basal Metabolic Rate

How many calories should you consume in any given day? And how many fewer do you need to consume in order to lose weight? In general terms, most men can lose weight on an 1,800-calorie diet; most women can lose weight on about 1,200. Obviously, this is a pretty blunt instrument, and one that doesn't account for variations in size and activity level. As a result, you may end up eating fewer calories than you need to lose weight—and that's no good. There's a better, more specific tool for determining how many calories you need to consume to make sure your body has the fuel it needs, while still allowing you to lose weight.

To determine your calorie needs, you need to use the Harris-Benedict equations, which gives you a number called your Basal Metabolic Rate (BMR), which essentially means the number of calories you burn simply by living. The equations might look a little harrowing for math phobics, but I'll walk you through them step by step, making it as simple as I can, so that you just have to plug in the numbers. (A calculator will certainly help.)

Step One: Determine Your Weight in Kilograms
Your weight in pounds divided by 2.2 = your weight in kilograms. (For example: 190 pounds divided by 2.2 = 86 kilograms.)

Step Two: Determine Your Height in Inches
First, we need your height in inches. There are twelve inches in a foot. (For example: if you're five feet eight inches, you're 68 inches tall.)

Step Three: Determine Your Height in Centimeters
Your height in inches x 2.54. (For example: If you're 68 inches tall, 68 x 2.54 = 173 centimeters.)

Great. The conversions are over. Now all you have to do is plug those numbers into the equations.

Step Four
If you're male: multiply your weight in kilograms (your answer to Step One) by 13.7. If you're female: multiply your weight in kilograms (your answer to Step One) by 9.6. (For example, 86 kilograms x 13.7 = 1,182.)

Step Five
If you're male: multiply your height in centimeters (your answer to Step Three) by 5. If you're female: multiply your height in centimeters (your answer to Step Three) by 1.8. (For example, 173 centimeters x 5 = 865.)

Step Six
If you're male: multiply your age in years by 6.8. If you're female: multiply your age in years by 4.7. (For example, 54 x 6.8 = 367.)

Step Seven
Add the following: 66 + your answer to Step Four + your answer to Step Five. (For example, 66 + 1,182 + 585 = 2,113.)

Step Eight
Subtract your answer to Step Six from your answer to Step Seven. (For example, 2,113 - 367 = 1,746.)

Your answer to Step Eight is your basal metabolic rate (BMR), and it represents the number of calories you need just to survive. In other words, that's the number of calories you'd burn during the day if you never even got out of bed. This is your baseline: you should not consume fewer calories than your BMR.

Of course, you need more fuel than that; even if you're relatively sedentary, you are burning more calories than your BMR as soon as you get up in the morning. But activity levels range widely, depending on what you do for a living and how often you exercise. The multiplier below will help you to calculate accurately the number of calories you require to get through a typical day, while maintaining your current weight.

Step Nine
Use this activity multiplier to determine approximately how many calories you really need in a day (remember, your BMR is your answer to Step Eight).

Sedentary (little or no exercise, desk job) = BMR x 1.2. Lightly active (light exercise 1 to 3 days a week) = BMR x 1.375. Moderately active (moderate exercise 3 to 5 days a week) = BMR x 1.55. Very active (hard exercise 6 to 7 days a week) = BMR x 1.725. Super active (hard daily exercise and a hard physical job, or 2 to 3 days a week of active training for an athletic event such as a marathon) = BMR x 1.9.

You answer to Step Nine is the number of calories you really need in a day. The next step, of course, is to determine how many calories you can eat and still lose weight.

Step Ten

Subtract 500 calories from your answer to Step Nine. This is your magic number, the number of calories that you can eat every day, and see a healthy, gradual weight loss—about a pound or two a week.

As you'll see, the model Chilton Program meal plans contain approximately 2,000 calories a day. I've included the calorie counts for the individual foods included in the plans so you can put together a version of the meal plans that works for your individual caloric needs. So if you need to lose weight, go back to Step Ten to determine the number of calories that you personally can eat in a day while losing weight. When you subtract that number from the 2,000 calories in the meal plans, you'll know how many calories you have to drop from the meal plans to make weight loss work for you. For instance, if you can lose weight at 1,800 calories, you'll need to cut 200 calories from the plans, which is easily accomplished by eliminating a snack. The only "fixed" item in the plans is the fish portion, which you should not cut, to ensure that you're getting the optimal balance of fatty acids.

For more details on a weight loss plan that individually fits you, go to the weight loss section at www.inflammationnation.com.

This at-a-glance table will enable you to make sure you keep your AA consumption within anti-inflammatory parameters. You'll arrive at your daily inflammatory index value by adding up the inflammatory index ratings of all the foods you've eaten that day.

◆ If you're following the Chilton Solution Plan, your total Inflammatory Index rating for the day should be under 100.

◆ If you're following the Chilton Prevention Plan, your total Inflammatory Index rating for the day should be under 150.

Some Notes on the Inflammatory Index

AA appears only in fish, meat, and in products derived from animals. For the purposes of this index, all other foods, such as fruit, vegetables, and grains, may be considered *free foods*.

The Inflammatory Index was determined using fatty-acid concentrations from the USDA Standard 13 and 16 databases. In many cases, the databases give several examples with corresponding fatty-acid levels for the same food. Often these values are different. Every effort has been made to approximate the average fatty-acid levels from all the examples provided in the databases.

Please note: the Inflammatory Index is as comprehensive as I could make it at this point in time, given the current information available. If you don't find the food for which you're looking, it's either because it contains little, or no, AA, or because the fatty-acid values for the food don't appear in the USDA databases. It is one of my hopes that this book will cause government organizations to better characterize a number of foods by taking AA levels into consideration.

Even a cursory glance at the Inflammatory Index will give you an idea of the major offenders, though. Foods with high levels of AA, or poor AA/EPA ratios, are those that contain mixed parts from livestock, organ meats, some farmed fish (salmon, in particular), eggs, and some poultry products (turkey, in particular).

I have broken the index up into Meat and Poultry, Fish, Dairy, Eggs, Fast Food, Baked Goods and Pasta, and Snacks.

MEAT AND POULTRY

FOOD	SERVING SIZE	INDEX VALUE	FOOD	SERVING SIZE	INDEX VALUE
Chitterlings	100 g	1,860	Chicken, thigh	100 g	100
Chicken, heart	100 g	720	Chicken, fat	100 g	100
Pork, liver	100 g	530	Pork sausage	100 g	90
Beef, brain	100 g	450	Veal	100 g	90
Chicken, giblets, fried	100 g	380	Moose	100 g	90
Chicken, liver	100 g	330	Bison	100 g	80
Beef, kidneys	100 g	330	Turkey, light meat	100 g	80
Turkey, liver	100 g	330	Lamb loin, lean	100 g	70
Bear meat	100 g	320	Turkey bologna	100 g	70
Pork, heart	100 g	310	Ostrich	100 g	70
Turkey, fat	100 g	300	Beerwurst	100 g	60
Veal, heart	100 g	280	Pork chops, oven fried	100 g	50
Turkey bacon	100 g	260	Chicken parmesan	100 g	50
Pâté de foie gras	100 g	250	Beef tenderloin, lean	100 g	40
Beef, liver	100 g	230	Beef, porterhouse	100 g	40
Chicken, stewed	100 g	200	Beef, T-bone	100 g	40
Quail	100 g	190	Beef, ribs	100 g	40
Salami (hard), pork	100 g	160	Pork tenderloin	100 g	40
Turkey, dark meat	100 g	160	Ham, sliced	100 g	40
Pork, cured bacon	100 g	150	Beef sausage	100 g	40
Cornish game hen	100 g	150	Hamburger (95% lean)	100 g	40
Turkey ham	100 g	140	Rib eye steak	100 g	40
Veal, bratwurst	100 g	130	Top sirloin	100 g	40
Bologna (chicken and pork)	100 g	110	Beef flank	100 g	30
Boar	100 g	110	Chicken pot pie	100 g	30
Chicken wings	100 g	110	USDA beef patties	100 g	30
Pork, cured ham	100 g	110	Pork skins	100 g	30
Chicken, fried	100 g	100	Bologna, beef	100 g	30
Chicken, leg	100 g	100	Deer, tenderloin	100 g	20

MEAT AND POULTRY (cont.)

FOOD	SERVING SIZE	INDEX VALUE	FOOD	SERVING SIZE	INDEX VALUE
Sausage and pepperoni pizza	100 g	20	Pepperoni pizza	100 g	10
Chili con carne	100 g	20	Pasta, meatballs, tomato sauce	100 g	10
Turkey breast, luncheon meat	100 g	20			

FISH

FOOD	SERVING SIZE	INDEX VALUE	FOOD	SERVING SIZE	INDEX VALUE
Atlantic salmon, farmed	100 g	150	Roe, mixed species	100 g	6
Atlantic salmon, wild	100 g	50	White tuna, canned	100 g	6
Channel catfish, wild	100 g	40	Chinook salmon	100 g	5
Sardine, Pacific	100 g	40	Pink salmon, wild	100 g	5
Channel catfish, farmed	100 g	40	Haddock	100 g	5
Flounder	100 g	30	Cod, Atlantic	100 g	5
Tuna salad	100 g	30	Atlantic mackerel, wild	100 g	4
Bass, freshwater	100 g	30	Scallops	100 g	4
Rainbow trout, wild	100 g	30	Smelt	100 g	4
Tilefish	100 g	20	Sockeye salmon	100 g	3
Walleye	100 g	20	Halibut, Greenland	100 g	3
Snapper, mixed species	100 g	20	Oysters, farmed	100 g	3
Swordfish	100 g	20	Alaskan king crab	100 g	2
Grouper	100 g	20	Chum salmon, wild	100 g	2
Shrimp, fried	100 g	20	Oysters, wild	100 g	2
Coho salmon, wild	100 g	10	Cod, Pacific	100 g	2
Blue crab	100 g	10	Herring, Atlantic	100 g	2
Clams	100 g	10	Rainbow trout, farmed	100 g	1
Mussels	100 g	10	Anchovy, European	100 g	1
Shark, mixed species	100 g	10	Seaweed, wakame	100 g	1
Octopus	100 g	10	Sea bass, mixed species	100 g	1
Perch, mixed species	100 g	9	Squid, mixed species	100 g	1
Caviar	100 g	8	Mahimahi	100 g	1
Yellowfin tuna, wild	100 g	7	Atlantic herring, wild	100 g	1

DAIRY

FOOD	SERVING SIZE	INDEX VALUE	FOOD	SERVING SIZE	INDEX VALUE
Cow's milk	100 g	0	Salad dressing, mayonnaise	100 g	20
Cheese, cow's milk	100 g	0			

EGGS

FOOD	SERVING SIZE	INDEX VALUE	FOOD	SERVING SIZE	INDEX VALUE
Egg yolk	100 g	340	Egg white	100 g	140
Duck egg	100 g	320	Egg salad	100 g	120

FAST FOOD

FOOD	SERVING SIZE	INDEX VALUE	FOOD	SERVING SIZE	INDEX VALUE
Chicken breaded, fried, dark meat	100 g	90	Biscuit with egg	100 g	50
Biscuit with egg and bacon	100 g	60	Biscuit with ham	100 g	30

BAKED GOODS AND PASTA

FOOD	SERVING SIZE	INDEX VALUE	FOOD	SERVING SIZE	INDEX VALUE
Cream puffs	100 g	50	Sweet roll	100 g	20
French toast	100 g	40	Coffee cake	100 g	20
Peanut-butter cookies	100 g	40	Pound cake	100 g	20
Doughnut	100 g	30	Egg custard	100 g	10
Eclair, custard pastry	100 g	30	Ice cream, vanilla	100 g	10
Waffles	100 g	20	Cheese cake	100 g	10
Yellow cake	100 g	20	Chocolate chip cookies	100 g	10
Brownies	100 g	20	Oatmeal cookies	100 g	10
Apple cinnamon danish	100 g	20	Vanilla wafers	100 g	10
Pancakes	100 g	20	Muffins	100 g	10
Banana cream pie	100 g	20	Dinner roll	100 g	10
Egg custard pie	100 g	20	Corn bread	100 g	10
Lemon meringue	100 g	20	Pasta made with egg	100 g	10

SNACKS

FOOD	SERVING SIZE	INDEX VALUE	FOOD	SERVING SIZE	INDEX VALUE
Peanuts	100 g	40	Potato pancakes	100 g	30
Potato sticks	100 g	30	Hush puppies	100 g	20

Source: USDA National Nutrient Database for Standard Reference Releases 13 and 16 (2003).

Chapter Fourteen

The Glycemic Ranking

The Glycemic Index (GI) is a measurement of how rapidly carbohydrates break down and affect the glucose level of the blood. Foods that break down more slowly are more desirable, because they do not cause a rapid spike of sugars in the blood—or the crash that inevitably follows.

Foods that break down slowly have a low-to-moderate rating on the Glycemic Index. The foods in these categories are the most appropriate choices for the Chilton Program.

> There are a number of Glycemic Index charts available, both on the Internet and in book form. Most assign white bread a GI value of 100 as their starting point. Values tend to vary slightly between them, so for the purposes of the Chilton Diet, I have simplified those into three lists: low, moderate, and high ratings on the Glycemic Index.
>
> If you wish to pursue more specific rankings, please note that I have used the following guidelines to create the lists below:
>
> Low GI: 55 or less
> Moderate GI: 56 to 69
> High GI: 70 and up

Foods That Rank Low on the Glycemic Index: *(Eat these foods often)*

Lentils, kidney beans, chickpeas, lima beans, split peas

Most fruits, including apples, fresh apricots, cherries, oranges, peaches, pears, plums, grapefruit, and strawberries

Nonstarchy vegetables, including artichokes, asparagus, beets, broccoli, brussel sprouts, cabbage, carrots, cauliflower, celery, cucumber, eggplant, green and yellow beans, leafy greens, lettuces (all kinds), spinach, mushrooms, peppers, tomatoes, zucchini and other summer squash

Pearled barley

Whole-wheat pasta

Nuts and peanuts

Milk, whole and skim

Low-fat yogurt

Foods That Rank Moderate on the Glycemic Index: *(Eat these foods in moderation)*

Yams, sweet potatoes

Corn

Canned beans

Peas

Slow-cooking oatmeal

Foods That Rank High on the Glycemic Index: *(Eat these foods very rarely; avoid them, if possible)*

Bread (unless whole-grain or a low-carbohydrate brand)

Cereals (unless a low-carbohydrate brand)

Crackers and pretzels

Popcorn

Corn chips

Instant rice

Instant oatmeal

Cookies

Cakes, muffins, doughnuts, danishes

Ice cream

Jams and jellies

Potatoes, turnips

Some fruits, including dates, raisins; canned fruits in syrup; tropical fresh fruit like kiwi, mango, papaya, watermelon, pineapple

Honey

Sugar (white and brown)

Maple syrup

Chapter Fifteen
The Chilton Fish Ranking

Fish will assume a starring role in your diet when you do the Chilton Program, but as you now know, not all fish are alike. Different fish have different ratios of beneficial and harmful fatty acids. For example, I looked at the ratios and concentrations of inflammatory AA to beneficial EPA, and I divided the fish options up into categories so that you can easily tell what your best and worst choices are.

Don't be confused if the Inflammatory Index value of a fish appears to conflict with that same fish's position on the list below. The Inflammatory Index allows you to determine the impact of AA in a food, without factoring in the impact of large amounts of beneficial EPA. The list below takes both into consideration.

Categories 1 and 2: I'd like you to eat as many of the fish types listed in Categories 1 and 2 as you possibly can. These contribute significantly to the amount of EPA that I recommend you get for the day, so if you eat these fish when recommended, you do not need to supplement with EPA.

Because fish fatty acids have a mild blood-thinning effect, they should not be combined with powerful blood-thinning medications such as Coumadin (warfarin) or heparin, except on a physician's advice.

Category 3: the fish types in Category 3 are neutral; these *do not* count toward your EPA needs for the day.

Category 4: the fish choices in this category contain high levels of AA, or ratios of AA to EPA of greater than 1, and should be avoided if possible.

> Note: In March 2004, the Food and Drug Administration recommended that pregnant women and young children avoid shark, swordfish, king mackerel, and tilefish because these large fish may contain unsafe levels of methylmercury. The administration further recommends that pregnant women restrict themselves to twelve ounces of fish a week.
>
> Oils from supplements are screened for mercury, but you should not take any supplement or medication if you are pregnant, except on the advice of your doctor or midwife.

Category 1 Fish: Best Fish *(These are your best choices: eat them as often as possible)*

Anchovies, European

Herring, Atlantic/Pacific

Mackerel, Atlantic/Pacific

Chinook salmon, wild

Roe, mixed species

Caviar, black and red

Sockeye salmon, wild

Category 2 Fish: Good Fish *(These are your good choices: eat them often)*

Pink salmon, wild

Halibut, Greenland

Coho salmon, wild

Alaskan king crab

Blue crab

Chum salmon, wild

Smelt

Shrimp

Oysters, wild

Oysters, farmed

Mussels

Shark, mixed species

Sea bass, mixed species

White tuna, canned

Squid, mixed species

Category 3 Fish: Neutral *(There's no reason to avoid these fish, but they do not satisfy your EPA requirements; when you eat one of them in place of a category 1 or 2 fish, you will have to include an EPA supplement)*

Scallops

Clams

Flounder

Rainbow trout, wild

Yellowfin tuna

Trout, mixed species

Swordfish

Walleye

Sardines, Pacific

Salmon, Atlantic, wild

Tilefish

Haddock

Cod, Pacific

Cod, Atlantic

Octopus

Perch, mixed species

Snapper, mixed species

Mahimahi

Category 4 Fish: Bad Fish *(These are the bad choices, high in AA: avoid them, if possible)*

Grouper

Halibut, Atlantic/Pacific

Pompano, Florida

Channel catfish, farmed

Channel catfish, wild

Salmon, Atlantic, farmed

Chapter Sixteen
The Chilton Prevention Diet

The Chilton Prevention Prescription

For people with a moderate risk of overactive inflammation.

- Eat foods whose values add up to no more than 150 on the Inflammatory Index per day.

- Eat an average of at least 200 milligrams a day of EPA. This equates to roughly three servings of Category 1 or 2 fish a week, or four servings of Category 3 fish. If you'd prefer to supplement instead, take one capsule (typically 150 to 180 milligrams) of EPA twice daily, with breakfast and dinner. This delivers more than I recommend, but remains within acceptable ratios.

- Take an average of at least 450 to 550 milligrams of GLA a day in supplement form, which means a capsule (typically about 210 to 240 milligrams) twice daily, with breakfast and dinner.

- DO NOT take the recommended doses of GLA without having EPA—either through the fish you're eating or by supplementation in your diet.

- Choose carbohydrates with a low-to-moderate Glycemic Index value.

DAY 1

BREAKFAST—Cottage Cheese with Strawberries, Oat-Bran Muffin with Margarine
½ cup 1% cottage cheese (81)
1 cup strawberries (53)
1 small low-fat oat-bran muffin (178)
1 teaspoon trans-fat-free margarine (9)

1 borage oil capsule (taken with meal) (9)

LUNCH—Oriental Flank Steak (221) with Orange Vinaigrette (132), Whole-Wheat Dinner Roll, Fresh Fruit Salad
Oriental Flank Steak with Orange Vinaigrette
2 cups green leaf lettuce (17)
3 ounces cooked beef flank steak (158)
¼ cup mandarin oranges (23)
¼ cup grated carrots (11)
¼ cup sliced red onion (12)
1 tablespoon peanut oil (119)
1 ounce orange juice (13)

1 small whole-wheat dinner roll (75)

Fresh Fruit Salad
⅓ cup kiwi (36)
⅓ cup grapes (36)
⅓ cup strawberries (18)

DINNER—Grilled Salmon Teriyaki (382)*, Green Beans Almandine (203), Brown Rice, Baked Apple
Grilled Salmon Teriyaki
6 ounces broiled or grilled sockeye salmon (or another Category 1 fish) (367)
1 tablespoon reduced-sodium teriyaki sauce (15)

Green Beans Almandine
1 cup cooked green beans (38)
2 tablespoons sliced almonds (78)
1 tablespoon trans-fat-free margarine (87)

1 cup cooked brown rice (216)
1 medium apple baked with cinnamon (72)

1 borage oil capsule (taken with meal) (9)

SNACK—Crackers with Cheese
8 whole-wheat crackers (142)
1 ounce low-fat cheese (98)

DAY 1 Nutritional Values
Calories—1970
Fiber (g)—31.18
GI = all<70
% Fat—35.62
% SFA—7.80
% MUFA—16.03
% PUFA—9.41
AA (mg)—80
EPA (mg)—900
Cholesterol (mg)—206

* You'll find recipes for items marked with an asterisk * in chapter 18.

Note. Parenthetical values indicate number of calories. Nutritional value abbreviations: GI, glycemic index; % Fat, % calories from fat; % SFA, % calories from saturated fatty acids; % MUFA, % calories from monounsaturated fatty acids; % PUFA, % calories from polyunsaturated fatty acids; AA, arachidonic acid; EPA, eicosapentaenoic acid.

DAY 2

BREAKFAST—Waffle with Margarine and Blueberries, Yogurt

1 (7-inch) round whole-wheat waffle (218)
1 cup blueberries (83)
1 teaspoon trans-fat-free margarine (29)
6 ounces sugar-free, nonfat yogurt (73)

1 borage oil capsule (taken with meal) (9)

LUNCH—Hawaiian Toast with Sliced Tomatoes

Hawaiian Toast
2 slices oat-bran bread (142)
2 teaspoons trans-fat-free margarine (58)
4 ounces lean ham (105)
½ cup pineapple (49)
2 ounces low-fat Swiss cheese (100)

1 large tomato, sliced (33)

DINNER—Beef Stroganoff (553) with Pasta and Carrots

Beef Stroganoff
6 ounces cooked lean beef top sirloin (332)
    sautéed with 1 tablespoon canola oil (120)
½ cup cooked mushrooms (20)
4 tablespoons low-fat sour cream (81)

1 cup cooked whole-wheat pasta (174)
1 cup cooked carrots (55)
1 teaspoon trans-fat-free margarine (29)

1 borage oil capsule (taken with meal) (9)

SNACK—Fresh Grapes

2 cups grapes (221)

DAY 2 Nutritional Values
Calories—1,940
Fiber (g)—26.82
GI = all<70
% Fat—33.35
% SFA—9.64
% MUFA—14.30
% PUFA—7.52
AA (mg)—130
EPA (mg)—0
Cholesterol (mg)—314

DAY 3

BREAKFAST—MultiGrain Cheerios with Milk and Dried Apricots, Grapefruit
1 cup MultiGrain Cheerios (180)
1 cup 1% milk (102)
4 dried apricot halves (34)
½ medium grapefruit (41)

1 borage oil capsule (taken with meal) (9)

LUNCH—Tuna Pasta Salad (503)*, Cucumber Salad, Fresh Apple
Tuna Pasta Salad
3 ounces canned white tuna (109)
1 cup cooked whole-wheat pasta (174)
2 tablespoons no-cholesterol mayonnaise dressing (206)
¼ cup diced celery (4)
¼ cup diced red bell peppers (10)

Cucumber Salad
¾ cup sliced cucumbers (11)
½ tablespoon canola oil (60)
Vinegar and herbs of choice

1 small apple (55)

DINNER—Grilled Pork Chop, Sweet Potato, Green Peas, Vanilla Pudding with Plums
4 ounces grilled or broiled top loin pork chop (194)
1 medium baked sweet potato (103)
¾ cup cooked green peas (94)
1 tablespoon trans-fat-free margarine (87)
1 cup sugar-free, nonfat vanilla pudding (151)
½ cup plum slices (38)

1 borage oil capsule (taken with meal) (9)

SNACK—Mixed Nuts
½ cup dry-roasted mixed nuts (407)

DAY 3 Nutritional Values
Calories—2,078
Fiber (g)—31.25
GI = all<70
% Fat—40.77
% SFA—6.88
% MUFA—18.39
% PUFA—12.78
AA (mg)—110
EPA (mg)—200
Cholesterol (mg)—133

* You'll find recipes for items marked with an asterisk * in chapter 18.

DAY 4

BREAKFAST—Oat-Bran Bagel with Cream Cheese, Yogurt, Cantaloupe
½ medium oat-bran bagel (73)
1 tablespoon low-fat cream cheese (35)
6 ounces sugar-free, nonfat yogurt (73)
1 cup cantaloupe (54)

1 borage oil capsule (taken with meal) (9)

LUNCH—Taco Salad with Ranch Dressing (474) and Tortilla Chips
Taco Salad with Low-Fat Ranch Dressing
2 cups lettuce (11)
4 ounces cooked ground beef
    (95% lean) (194)
½ cup chopped tomatoes (16)
¼ cup chopped onion (12)
2 tablespoons canned black beans (27)
2 tablespoons corn kernels (79)
½ ounce low-fat cheese (25)
3 tablespoons low-fat ranch dressing (110)

1 ounce low-fat tortilla chips (132)

DINNER—Shrimp-and-Vegetable Stir-Fry I* (610), Tossed Green Salad with Vinaigrette Dressing, Roll with Margarine

Shrimp and Vegetable Stir-Fry I
5 ounces cooked shrimp (140)
½ cup chopped celery (8)
½ cup chopped green pepper (15)
½ cup diced tomatoes (34)
2 tablespoons olive oil to sauté shrimp and
    vegetables (239)
1 cup cooked whole-wheat pasta (174)

Tossed Green Salad with
Vinaigrette Dressing
1 cup green leaf lettuce (8)
3 cherry tomatoes (9)
2 tablespoons vinegar and olive oil salad
    dressing (144)

1 medium whole-wheat dinner roll (96)
1 teaspoon trans-fat-free margarine (29)

1 borage oil capsule (taken with meal) (9)

SNACK—Crackers with Cheese and Apple Slices
6 whole-wheat crackers (106)
2 ounces low-fat cheese (98)
1 small apple, sliced (55)

DAY 4 Nutritional Values
Calories—2014
Fiber (g)—30.15
GI = all<70
% Fat—37.88
% SFA—8.79
% MUFA—17.86
% PUFA—9.08
AA (mg)—160
EPA (mg)—240
Cholesterol (mg)—400

* You'll find recipes for items marked with an asterisk * in chapter 18.

DAY 5

BREAKFAST—Scrambled Egg Substitutes, Canadian Bacon, Toast with Margarine, Tomato Juice

½ cup cooked liquid egg substitute (105)
1 ounce Canadian bacon (45)
2 slices whole-wheat bread (138)
2 teaspoons trans-fat-free margarine (58)
6 ounces tomato juice (31)

1 borage oil capsule (taken with meal) (9)

LUNCH—Italian Chicken Sandwich (445), Tossed Salad with Italian Dressing, Fresh Grapes

Italian Chicken Sandwich
2 slices whole-wheat bread (138)
2 ounces cooked chicken breast (no skin) (98), sautéed in 1 tablespoon olive oil (119)
2 tablespoons marinara sauce (18)
1 ounce part-skim mozzarella cheese (72)

Tossed Salad with Italian Dressing
1 cup green leaf lettuce (8)
4 cherry tomatoes (12)
2 tablespoons grated carrots (6)
2 tablespoons Italian dressing (86)

1 cup grapes (110)

DINNER—Beef Short Ribs, Yellow Corn, Steamed Broccoli, Roll with Margarine, Waldorf-Gelatin Salad (121)

6 ounces cooked lean beef short ribs (405)
1 cup cooked corn (177)
1 cup cooked broccoli (44)
1 ounce whole-wheat dinner roll (75)
1 teaspoon trans-fat-free margarine (29)

Sugar-Free Waldorf-Gelatin Salad
½ cup sugar-free gelatin (9)
¼ small apple, chopped (14)
2 tablespoons diced celery (2)
2 tablespoons English walnuts (96)

1 borage oil capsule (taken with meal) (9)

SNACK—Fresh Pear

1 medium pear (96)

DAY 5 Nutritional Values
Calories—2,009
Fiber (g)—29.71
GI = all<70
% Fat—38.66
% SFA—9.95
% MUFA—16.04
% PUFA—9.72
AA (mg)—120
EPA (mg)—10
Cholesterol (mg)—220

DAY 6

BREAKFAST—Oatmeal with Pecans and Bananas, Mozzarella Cheese Stick

1 cup cooked oatmeal (145)
2 tablespoons chopped pecans (94)
1 small banana (90)
1 ounce part-skim mozzarella
    cheese stick (86)

1 borage oil capsule (taken with meal) (9)

LUNCH—Salmon Cake* with Aioli (540), Corn-and-Black-Bean Salad (482)

Salmon Cake with Aioli
3 ounces canned pink salmon (118)
2 tablespoons plain bread crumbs (53)
2 tablespoons cooked liquid egg
    substitute (26)
2 tablespoons canola oil to fry salmon
    cake (240)
1 teaspoon no-cholesterol mayonnaise
    mixed with garlic and herbs of choice
    (103)

Corn-and-Black-Bean Salad
½ cup corn (303)
½ cup black beans (109)
¼ cup chopped red peppers (10)
½ tablespoon canola oil (60)
Vinegar, lemon juice, cilantro,
    and spices of choice

DINNER—Baked Ham, Cabbage, Carrots, Applesauce

6 ounces smoked or cured lean baked
    ham (247)
1 cup cooked cabbage (33)
¾ cup cooked carrots (41)
½ tablespoon trans-fat-free margarine (43)
¾ cup unsweetened applesauce (79)

1 borage oil capsule (taken with meal) (9)

SNACK—Yogurt Crunch

8 ounces sugar-free nonfat yogurt (98)
2 tablespoons Fiber One cereal (15)

DAY 6 Nutritional Values
Calories—2,011
Fiber (g)—35.76
GI = all<70
% Fat—40.35
% SFA—7.26
% MUFA—18.12
% PUFA—13.25
AA (mg)—70
EPA (mg)—720
Cholesterol (mg)—157

* You'll find recipes for items marked with an asterisk * in chapter 18.

DAY 7

BREAKFAST—Peanut-Butter-and-Jelly Sandwich (402), Milk

Peanut-Butter-and-Jelly Sandwich
2 slices oat-bran bread (142)
2 tablespoons peanut butter (192)
2 tablespoons reduced- or no-sugar
  jelly (68)

1 cup 1% milk (102)

1 borage oil capsule (taken with meal) (9)

LUNCH—Meatball Hoagie (423), Tossed Salad with Vinaigrette Dressing, Strawberries

Meatball Hoagie
1 small whole-wheat hoagie roll (173)
3 ounces cooked ground beef
  (95% lean) (145)
½ cup sliced onions (24)
¼ cup sliced green peppers (5)
1 teaspoon canola oil to sauté vegetables
  (40)
¼ cup marinara sauce (36)

Tossed Salad with Vinaigrette Dressing
1 cup lettuce (6)
3 cherry tomatoes (9)
1 tablespoon olive oil with vinegar and herbs
  of choice (119)

1½ cups strawberries (69)

DINNER—Chicken Salsa (330), Spanish Rice (125), Green Beans, Corn Bread with Margarine

Chicken Salsa
4 ounces chicken breast (no skin) (196)
½ cup salsa (36)
2 ounces low-fat Cheddar cheese (98)

Spanish Rice
½ cup cooked brown rice (108)
¼ cup diced tomatoes (17)

1 cup cooked green beans (38)

1 ounce corn bread (prepared from mix) (89)
2 tablespoons trans-fat-free margarine (173)

1 borage oil capsule (taken with meal) (9)

SNACK—Pretzels

1 ounce whole-wheat pretzels (103)

DAY 7 Nutritional Values
Calories—2,006
Fiber (g)—29.10
GI = all<70
% Fat—37.65
% SFA—8.92
% MUFA—18.93
% PUFA—8.40
AA (mg)—140
EPA (mg)—10
Cholesterol (mg)—202

DAY 8

BREAKFAST—Cheese Omelet (154), Toast with Margarine, Citrus Sections
Cheese Omelet
½ cup cooked liquid egg substitute (105)
1 ounce low-fat cheese (49)

2 slices whole-wheat bread (138)
2 teaspoons trans-fat-free margarine (58)
½ cup grapefruit sections (37)
½ cup orange sections (42)

1 borage oil capsule (taken with meal) (9)

LUNCH—Shrimp Chowder* (527), Whole-Wheat Roll, Fresh Melon
Shrimp Chowder
4 ounces cooked shrimp (112)
1 cup 1% milk (102)
2 tablespoons trans-fat-free margarine (173)
2 tablespoons whole-wheat flour (51)
½ cup cooked corn (89)

1 small whole-wheat roll (75)

½ cup honeydew melon (32)
½ cup cantaloupe (30)

DINNER—Barbeque Pork Roast, Kidney Beans, Summer Squash, Chocolate Banana Parfait (164)
3 ounces lean pork shoulder roast (197)
    cooked with 2 tablespoons barbecue
    sauce (12)
½ cup cooked kidney beans (104)
1 cup summer squash (36), sautéed in
    2 teaspoons canola oil (80)

Chocolate Banana Parfait
½ cup sugar-free, nonfat chocolate
    pudding (74)
1 small banana (90)

1 borage oil capsule (taken with meal) (9)

SNACK—Crackers with Artificial Crab Salad (194)
6 whole-wheat crackers (106)

Artificial Crab Salad (194)
3 ounces imitation crabmeat (surimi) (87)
1 tablespoon no-cholesterol mayonnaise
    dressing (103)
¼ cup diced celery (4)

DAY 8 Nutritional Values
Calories—2,004
Fiber (g)—27.89
GI = all<70
% Fat—36.73
% SFA—8.15
% MUFA—15.04
% PUFA—11.14
AA (mg)—140
EPA (mg)—400
Cholesterol (mg)—330

---

* You'll find recipes for items marked with an asterisk * in chapter 18.

DAY 9

BREAKFAST—Shredded-Wheat Cereal with Milk and Blueberries, Orange Juice
1 cup bite-sized shredded-wheat cereal (167)
1 cup 1% milk (102)
1 cup blueberries (83)
6 ounces unsweetened orange juice (78)

1 borage oil capsule (taken with meal) (9)

LUNCH—Chicken-and-White-Bean Salad (390), Baby Carrots
Chicken-and-White-Bean Salad
3 ounces cooked chicken breast (no skin) (147)
⅓ cup canned white beans (101)
2 tablespoons cooked green peas (14)
2 tablespoons chopped sweet red peppers (5)
2 tablespoons chopped green onions (4)
1 tablespoon olive oil (119)
Vinegar, lemon juice, and herbs as desired

5 baby carrots (18)

DINNER—Spaghetti and Meatballs (498), Tomato-and-Mozzarella Salad (223), Tuscan Ricotta with Nuts and Fruit (282)
1½ cups cooked whole-wheat spaghetti (260)
3 ounces cooked ground beef (95% lean) (145)
½ cup marinara sauce (71)
1 tablespoon grated Parmesan cheese (22)

Tomato-and-Mozzarella Salad
1 cup chopped fresh tomatoes (32)
1 ounce part-skim mozzarella cheese (72)
1 tablespoon olive oil (119)
Balsamic vinegar and chopped fresh basil

Tuscan Ricotta with Nuts and Fruit
½ cup part-skim ricotta cheese (170)
2 tablespoons sliced almonds (78)
4 dried apricot halves (34)

1 borage oil capsule (taken with meal) (9)

SNACK—Celery Stuffed with Low-Fat Cream Cheese
2 celery stalks (11)
4 tablespoons low-fat cream cheese (139)

DAY 9 Nutritional Values
Calories—2,009
Fiber (g)—33.45
GI = all<70
% Fat—34.72
% SFA—12.24
% MUFA—17.24
% PUFA—3.92
AA (mg)—110
EPA (mg)—10
Cholesterol (mg)—243

DAY 10

BREAKFAST—Scrambled Egg Substitute, English Muffin with Margarine and Jelly, Tomato Juice
½ cup cooked liquid egg substitute (105)
1 whole-wheat English muffin (134)
2 teaspoons trans-fat-free margarine (58)
2 tablespoons reduced- or no-sugar jelly (68)
8 ounces tomato juice (41)

1 borage oil capsule (taken with meal) (9)

LUNCH—Cheeseburger (309), Cucumber-and-Tomato Salad (84), Fresh Apple
Cheeseburger
1 multigrain hamburger roll (113)
3 ounces cooked ground beef (95% lean) (145)
1 ounce low-fat cheese (49)
1 lettuce leaf (2)

Cucumber-and-Tomato Salad
¼ cup sliced cucumber (4)
¼ cup chopped tomato (8)
1 tablespoon vinegar and oil salad dressing (72)

1 medium apple (72)

DINNER—Lemon-Herb Mackerel*
(or another Category 1 fish), Baked Brown Rice (295), Broccoli Parmesan (155), Roll with Margarine
4 ounces broiled or grilled mackerel (or another Category 1 fish) (297)
Lemon juice and herbs of choice

Baked Brown Rice
¾ cup cooked brown rice (162)
¼ cup grated cooked carrots (14)
1 tablespoon olive oil (119)

Broccoli Parmesan
1 cup cooked broccoli (44)
1 ounce Parmesan cheese (111)

1 ounce whole-wheat roll (75)
½ tablespoon trans-fat-free margarine (43)

1 borage oil capsule (taken with meal) (9)

SNACK—Banana Milk Shake (251)
Banana Milk Shake
½ cup 1% milk (51)
½ cup sugar-free, nonfat frozen yogurt (100)
¾ cup sliced banana (100)

DAY 10 Nutritional Values
Calories—2,005
Fiber (g)—27.28
GI = all<70
% Fat—36.96
% SFA—10.28
% MUFA—16.44
% PUFA—8.33
AA (mg)—100
EPA (mg)—570
Cholesterol (mg)—186

---

* You'll find recipes for items marked with an asterisk * in chapter 18.

DAY 11

BREAKFAST—Oat-Bran Bagel with Cream Cheese, Apple Juice
1 medium oat-bran bagel (181)
2 tablespoons low-fat cream cheese (69)
6 ounces unsweetened apple juice (87)

1 borage oil capsule (taken with meal) (9)

LUNCH—Hawaiian Pizza Salad with Vinaigrette Dressing, Crackers, Grapes
Hawaiian Pizza Salad with Vinaigrette Dressing
2 cups green leaf lettuce (17)
3 ounces extra-lean ham (110)
2 ounces part-skim mozzarella cheese (144)
¼ cup diced pineapple (19)
½ cup diced fresh tomatoes (13)
2 tablespoons vinegar and oil salad dressing (144)

5 whole-wheat crackers (89)
2 cups grapes (221)

DINNER—Grilled Beef Tenderloin, Cauliflower with Cheese (78), Green Peas, Pears
6 ounces grilled or broiled beef tenderloin (359)

Cauliflower with Cheese
1 cup cooked cauliflower (29)
1 ounce low-fat Cheddar cheese (49)

1 cup cooked green peas (125)
1 teaspoon trans-fat-free margarine (29)
1 cup pear slices (71)

1 borage oil capsule (taken with meal) (9)

SNACK—Pistachio Nuts
½ cup dry-toasted pistachio nuts (231)

DAY 11 Nutritional Values
Calories—2,005
Fiber (g)—30.85
GI = all<70
% Fat—36.52
% SFA—11.45
% MUFA—14.10
% PUFA—8.36
AA (mg)—70
EPA (mg)—0
Cholesterol (mg)—241

DAY 12

BREAKFAST—Bran Muffin with Margarine, Cottage Cheese with Peaches
1 medium low-fat bran muffin (169)
2 teaspoons trans-fat-free margarine (58)
¾ cup 1% cottage cheese (122)
½ cup peaches (29)

1 borage oil capsule (taken with meal) (9)

LUNCH—Cobb Shrimp Salad with Ranch Dressing (515), Roll with Margarine, Frozen Yogurt
Cobb Shrimp Salad with Low-Fat
Ranch Dressing
2 cups green leaf lettuce (17)
4 ounces cooked shrimp (112)
1 slice cooked lean bacon (37)
¼ cup chopped tomatoes (7)
2 tablespoons cooked corn (76)
¼ cup grated carrots (11)
½ cup avocado (120)
¼ cup low-fat ranch salad dressing (135)

1 small whole-wheat roll (75)
½ tablespoon trans-fat-free margarine (43)

1 cup sugar-free nonfat frozen yogurt (199)

DINNER—Barbeque Chicken (219), Corn on the Cob, Coleslaw (133), Cherries
4 ounces chicken breast (no skin) (196),
    cooked with 2 tablespoons barbecue
    sauce (23)
1 ear corn (83) with 1 tablespoon trans-fat-
    free margarine (87)

Coleslaw
1 cup chopped cabbage (21)
2 tablespoons low-fat coleslaw
    dressing (112)

¾ cup cherries (55)

1 borage oil capsule (taken with meal) (9)

SNACK—Yogurt with Peaches and Almonds
8 ounces sugar-free, nonfat yogurt (98)
1 medium peach (38)
2 tablespoons sliced almonds (69)

DAY 12 Nutritional Values
Calories—2,010
Fiber (g)—28.19
GI = all<70
% Fat—35.52
% SFA—6.71
% MUFA—16.32
% PUFA—9.34
AA (mg)—190
EPA (mg)—210
Cholesterol (mg)—388

DAY 13

BREAKFAST—Muesli Cereal with Milk, Waffles with Margarine and Apples, Cranapple Juice
¾ cup muesli cereal (217)
1 cup 1% milk (102)
1 (7-inch) round whole-wheat waffle (218)
2 teaspoons trans-fat-free margarine (58)
½ cup apples (73)
4 ounces sugar-free cranapple juice (23)

1 borage oil capsule (taken with meal) (9)

LUNCH—Chicken Salad Sandwich (520), Fruit Salad
Chicken Salad Sandwich
1 whole-wheat sandwich roll (114)
4 ounces cooked chicken breast (no skin) (196)
¼ cup chopped celery (4)
2 tablespoons no-cholesterol mayonnaise dressing (206)

¼ cup peaches (17)
¼ cup blueberries (21)
¼ cup grapes (28)
¼ cup kiwi (27)

DINNER—Crabmeat Lasagna Rolls* (341), Sautéed Zucchini, Spinach Salad with Vinaigrette Dressing (83)
Crabmeat Lasagna Roll
2 ounces whole-wheat lasagna noodles, cooked (74)
4 ounces canned blue-crab meat (112)
¼ cup 1% cottage cheese (41)
2 tablespoons grated Parmesan cheese (43)
½ cup marinara sauce (71)

1 cup zucchini (29), sautéed with 1 teaspoon olive oil (40) and herbs of choice

Spinach Salad with Vinaigrette Dressing
1 cup fresh spinach (7)
¼ cup sliced mushrooms (4)
¼ cup sliced red onions (12)

½ tablespoon olive oil (60)
Vinegar and herbs of choice

1 borage oil capsule (taken with meal) (9)

SNACK—Ham-and-Cheese Finger Sandwiches (186)
Ham-and-Cheese Finger Sandwiches
1 slice mixed-grain bread (65)
1 ounce extra-lean ham (37)
1 ounce low-fat cheese (50)
1 teaspoon no-cholesterol mayonnaise dressing (34)

DAY 13 Nutritional Values
Calories—2,001
Fiber (g)—23.54
GI = all<70
% Fat—36.03
% SFA—7.78
% MUFA—13.30
% PUFA—13.29
AA (mg)—180
EPA (mg)—230
Cholesterol (mg)—295

* You'll find recipes for the items marked with an asterisk* in chapter 18.

DAY 14

BREAKFAST—Swiss Cheese Toast (296) Grapefruit

Swiss Cheese Toast

2 slices whole-wheat bread (138)

2 teaspoons trans-fat-free margarine (58)

2 ounces low-fat Swiss cheese (100)

½ medium grapefruit (41)

1 borage oil capsule (taken with meal) (9)

LUNCH—Barbeque Pork Sandwich (389), Vinaigrette Coleslaw (81), Blackberry Crumble

Barbeque Pork Sandwich

1 whole-grain hamburger roll (114)

4 ounces roasted lean pork shoulder (263)

1 tablespoon barbeque sauce (12)

Vinaigrette Coleslaw

1 cup chopped cabbage (21)

½ tablespoon canola oil (60)

Artificial sweetener, vinegar, dill seed, and herbs of choice

Blackberry Crumble

1 cup blackberries (62)

2 tablespoons oats (76)

2 tablespoons sliced almonds (66)

DINNER—Steak Fajitas (511), Refried Beans, Guacamole Salad (134)

Steak Fajitas

4 ounces cooked beef flank steak (211)

½ cup sliced green peppers (9)

½ cup sliced red peppers (12)

½ cup sliced onions (24)

½ tablespoon canola oil to sauté steak and vegetables (60)

2 (6-inch) flour tortillas (195)

½ cup canned refried beans (118)

Guacamole Salad

½ cup lettuce (3)

½ cup chopped tomatoes (11)

½ cup avocado (120)

1 borage oil capsule (taken with meal) (9)

SNACK—Special K Cereal with Milk and Banana

½ cup Kellogg's Special K cereal (59)

¾ cup 1% milk (77)

1 small banana (72)

DAY 14 Nutritional Values

Calories—2,000

Fiber (g)—41.44

GI = all<70

% Fat—35.93

% SFA—9.11

% MUFA—17.96

% PUFA—6.68

AA (mg)—100

EPA (mg)—0

Cholesterol (mg)—191

DAY 15

**BREAKFAST—Mushroom-and-Spinach
Frittata (178), Toast with Margarine
Cantaloupe**
Mushroom-and-Spinach Frittata
½ cup cooked liquid egg substitute (105)
½ cup sliced mushrooms (8)
¼ cup chopped spinach (15)
1 ounce low-fat cheese (50)

1 slice whole-wheat bread (69)
1 teaspoon trans-fat-free margarine (29)
⅛ fresh cantaloupe (23)

1 borage oil capsule (taken with meal) (9)

**LUNCH—Chef's Salad with Ranch Dressing
(406), Crackers, Tropical Gelatin Salad (87)**
Chef's Salad with Low-Fat Ranch Dressing
2 cups lettuce (11)
5 cherry tomatoes (15)
¼ cup sliced cucumber (4)
¼ cup sliced mushrooms (4)
2 ounces lean ham (92)
2 ounces low-fat cheese (98)
1 ounce turkey breast (97% lean) (27)
4 large ripe olives (20)
¼ cup low-fat ranch salad dressing (135)

8 whole-wheat crackers (142)

Sugar-Free Tropical Gelatin Salad
1 cup sugar-free gelatin (19)
¼ cup mandarin oranges (23)
2 tablespoons chopped pecans (45)

**DINNER—Mackerel-and-Crab
Jambalaya* (591), Broccoli,
Whole-Wheat Roll with Margarine**
Mackerel-and-Crab Jambalaya
3 ounces cooked Atlantic mackerel
   (or another Category 1 fish) (223)
2 ounces cooked Alaskan king
   crab meat (55)
¼ cup chopped green peppers (5)
¼ cup chopped onions (17)

¼ cup chopped yellow peppers (7)
1 cup diced tomatoes (68)

1 cup cooked brown rice (216)

1 cup cooked broccoli (44)
1 medium whole-wheat roll (173)
1½ tablespoons trans-fat-free margarine
   (130)

1 borage oil capsule (taken with meal) (9)

SNACK—Peach Raspberry Smoothie (105)
Peach Raspberry Smoothie
6 ounces sugar-free nonfat yogurt (73)
¼ cup sliced peaches (16)
¼ cup raspberries (16)

DAY 15 Nutritional Values
Calories—1,995
Fiber (g)—33.00
GI = all<70
% Fat—35.00
% SFA—7.70
% MUFA—14.52
% PUFA—9.11
AA (mg)—90
EPA (mg)—600
Cholesterol (mg)—179

* You'll find recipes for items marked with an asterisk * in chapter 18.

DAY 16

BREAKFAST—English Muffin with Almond Butter, Orange, Milk

1 mixed-grain English muffin (155)

2 tablespoons almond butter (203)

1 medium orange (62)

1 cup 1% milk (102)

1 borage oil capsule (taken with meal) (9)

LUNCH—Chicken Club Sandwich (520), Fresh Apple

Chicken Club Sandwich

2 slices whole-wheat bread (138)

3 ounces cooked chicken breast (no skin) (147)

1 ounce low-fat cheese (50)

2 slices cooked lean bacon (74)

1 leaf lettuce (1)

2 slices tomato (7)

1 tablespoon no-cholesterol mayonnaise (103)

1 small apple (55)

DINNER—Vegetable-and-Tofu Stir-Fry (376), Pasta, Sweet Potatoes

Vegetable-and-Tofu Stir-Fry

4 ounces firm silken tofu (70)

1 cup sliced carrots (55)

½ cup snow peas (42)

½ cup chopped broccoli (22)

½ cup sliced mushrooms (22)

½ cup sliced onions (46)

1 tablespoon peanut oil to stir-fry tofu and vegetables (119)

1 cup cooked whole-wheat pasta (174)

½ cup cooked sweet potato (125)

1 teaspoon trans-fat-free margarine (29)

1 borage oil capsule (taken with meal) (9)

SNACK—Low-Fat Cheese and Crackers

5 whole-wheat crackers (89)

2 ounces low-fat cheese (98)

DAY 16 Nutritional Values

Calories—2,006

Fiber (g)—36.27

GI = all<70

% Fat—34.46

% SFA—7.48

% MUFA—14.79

% PUFA—10.36

AA (mg)—90

EPA (mg)—10

Cholesterol (mg)—124

DAY 17

BREAKFAST—Oatmeal with Peaches, Yogurt
1 cup cooked oatmeal (145)
1 small peach (31)
8 ounces sugar-free nonfat yogurt (98)

1 borage oil capsule (taken with meal) (9)

LUNCH—Seafood Pasta Salad* (603), Crackers, Berries
Seafood Pasta Salad
2 ounces canned blue crab (56)
2 ounces cooked shrimp (56)
1 cup cooked shell pasta (162)
½ cup cooked asparagus (20)
3 tablespoons no-cholesterol
   mayonnaise (309)

5 whole-wheat crackers (89)
½ cup strawberries (27)
½ cup blueberries (41)

DINNER—Beef Tenderloin with Béarnaise Sauce (424), Lemon Couscous, Brussels Sprouts
Beef Tenderloin with Béarnaise Sauce
5 ounces cooked lean beef tenderloin (299)
⅛ packet béarnaise sauce mix (12)
1 tablespoon trans-fat-free margarine (87)
¼ cup 1% milk (26)

Lemon Couscous
1 cup couscous, cooked with lemon juice
   and lemon zest added (176)

1 cup cooked brussels sprouts (56)
1 tablespoon trans-fat-free margarine (87)

1 borage oil capsule (taken with meal) (9)

SNACK—Fresh Grapes and Low-Fat Cheese
1 cup grapes (110)
2 ounces low-fat cheese (98)

DAY 17 Nutritional Values
Calories—2,003
Fiber (g)—21.65
GI = all<70
% Fat—37.90
% SFA—8.69
% MUFA—12.88
% PUFA—13.83
AA (mg)—140
EPA (mg)—210
Cholesterol (mg)—300

* You'll find recipes for items marked with an asterisk * in chapter 18.

DAY 18

BREAKFAST—Scrambled Egg Substitute, Canadian Bacon, Toast with Margarine and Jelly, Tomato Juice
½ cup cooked liquid egg substitute (105)
1 ounce Canadian-style bacon (45)
2 slices whole-wheat bread (138)
2 teaspoons trans-fat-free margarine (58)
1 tablespoons reduced- or no-sugar
    jelly (34)
8 ounces tomato juice (41)

1 borage oil capsule (taken with meal) (9)

LUNCH—Cucumber Soup, Rye Cracker, Roast Beef Sandwich (345)
Cucumber Soup
1 cup chopped cucumber (16)
¼ cup low-fat sour cream (82)
¼ cup condensed cream of chicken soup (58)

1 rye wafer (84)

Roast Beef Sandwich
3 ounces lean cooked eye of round
    beef (143)
2 slices multigrain bread (130)
1 teaspoon prepared horseradish (3)
2 teaspoons no-cholesterol mayonnaise (69)

DINNER—Shrimp-and-Scallops Scampi* (302), Green Beans, Risotto Primavera (389), Dinner Roll with Margarine
Shrimp-and-Scallops Scampi
3 ounces scallops (95)
3 ounces shrimp (84)
1 teaspoon chopped garlic (4)
1 tablespoon olive oil to sauté scallops
    and shrimp (119)

1 cup cooked green beans (38)

Risotto Primavera
½ cup chicken broth (39)
¾ cup cooked brown rice (162)
⅓ cup cooked snow peas (27)
⅛ cup chopped sweet red peppers (5)
⅓ cup chopped asparagus (13)

1 tablespoon trans-fat-free margarine, 70%
    vegetable oil spread (87)
½ ounce Parmesan cheese (56)

1 small whole-wheat roll (75)

1 borage oil capsule (taken with meal) (9)

SNACK—Cherry Crumble (183)
Cherry Crumble
1 cup cherries (74)
2 tablespoons oats (76)
1 tablespoon sliced almonds (33)

DAY 18 Nutritional Values
Calories—2,011
Fiber (g)—30.52
GI = all<70
% Fat—37.02
% SFA—9.45
% MUFA—16.78
% PUFA—8.71
AA (mg)—100
EPA (mg)—250
Cholesterol (mg)—325

* You'll find recipes for items marked with an asterisk * in chapter 18.

DAY 19

BREAKFAST—Peanut-Butter-and-Jelly Sandwich (360), Fresh Apple

Peanut-Butter-and-Jelly Sandwich

2 slices of whole-wheat bread (138)

2 tablespoons peanut butter (188)

1 tablespoon reduced- or no-sugar jelly (34)

1 medium apple (72)

1 borage oil capsule (taken with meal) (9)

LUNCH—Hot Dog on Bun, Macaroni Salad, Chocolate Pudding

1 beef frankfurter (148)

1 mixed-grain frankfurter roll (148)

1 teaspoon yellow mustard (3)

Macaroni Salad

1 cup cooked macaroni (197)

2 tablespoons diced celery (2)

2 tablespoons no-cholesterol mayonnaise (206)

½ cup sugar-free, nonfat chocolate pudding (74)

DINNER—Herbed-Pork Tenderloin, Cauliflower with Cheese Sauce (233), Snow Peas, Dinner Roll with Margarine

6 ounces cooked pork tenderloin rubbed with rosemary, pepper, and garlic salt (279)

Cauliflower with Cheese Sauce

1½ cups cooked cauliflower (43)

¼ cup white sauce (92)

2 ounces low-fat Cheddar cheese (98)

1 cup cooked snow peas (83)

1 small oat-bran dinner roll (67)

1 teaspoon trans-fat-free margarine (29)

1 borage oil capsule (taken with meal) (9)

SNACK—Fresh Pear

1 small pear (81)

DAY 19 Nutritional Values
Calories—2,000
Fiber (g)—29.42
GI = all<70
% Fat—38.75
% SFA—9.76
% MUFA—14.63
% PUFA—11.53
AA (mg)—50
EPA (mg)—0
Cholesterol (mg)—175

DAY 20

BREAKFAST—Multi-Bran Chex Cereal with Milk and Blueberries, Bagel with Cream Cheese

1 cup Multi-Bran Chex (166)
1 cup 1% milk (102)
½ cup blueberries (41)
½ medium oat-bran bagel (73)
1 tablespoon low-fat cream cheese (35)

1 borage oil capsule (taken with meal) (9)

LUNCH—Tuna Melt Sandwich* (467), Cucumber Salad (56), Frozen Yogurt
Tuna Melt Sandwich
1 mixed-grain English muffin (155)
3 ounces canned white tuna (109)
1 tablespoon no-cholesterol mayonnaise
    dressing (103)
2 ounces reduced-fat Swiss cheese (100)

Cucumber Salad
1 cup sliced cucumber (16)
1 teaspoon canola oil (40)
Vinegar, herbs, and spices of choice

1 cup sugar-free, nonfat frozen yogurt (199)

DINNER—Chopped Steak, Acorn Squash, Asparagus, Baked Apple
5 ounces cooked ground beef
    (95% lean) (242)
1 cup cooked acorn squash (83)
1 teaspoon trans-fat-free margarine (29)
1 cup cooked asparagus (40)
1 small apple (55)

1 borage oil capsule (taken with meal) (9)

SNACK—Mixed Nuts
½ cup dry-roasted mixed nuts (407)

DAY 20 Nutritional Values
Calories—2,013
Fiber (g)—34.31
GI = all<70
% Fat—35.37
% SFA—8.63
% MUFA—16.67
% PUFA—8.95
AA (mg)—120
EPA (mg)—200
Cholesterol (mg)—191

* You'll find recipes for items marked with an asterisk * in chapter 18.

DAY 21

BREAKFAST—Cheese Omelet (154), Toast with Margarine and Jelly, Orange Juice
Cheese Omelet
½ cup cooked liquid egg substitute (105)
1 ounce low-fat cheese (49)

2 slices multigrain bread (130)
2 teaspoons trans-fat-free margarine (58)
2 tablespoons reduced- or no-sugar
  jelly (68)
6 ounces unsweetened orange juice (78)

1 borage oil capsule (taken with meal) (9)

LUNCH—Chicken Salad (254), Crackers, Baby Carrots, Strawberries
Chicken Salad
3 ounces cooked chicken breast
  (no skin) (147)
1 tablespoon no-cholesterol
  mayonnaise (103)
¼ cup diced celery (4)

8 whole-wheat crackers (142)
6 baby carrots (21)
1 cup strawberries (53)

DINNER—Crab Cakes* (538), Broiled Tomato, Broccoli, Roll with Margarine
Crab Cakes
6 ounces Alaskan king crab meat (165)
2 tablespoons cooked liquid egg
  substitute (26)
¼ cup dry bread crumbs (107)
2 tablespoons canola oil to fry crab
  cakes (240)

1 medium tomato (22), broiled with
  ½ ounce grated Parmesan cheese (61)
1 cup cooked broccoli (44)
1 small whole-wheat dinner roll (75)
1 teaspoon trans-fat-free margarine (29)

1 borage oil capsule (taken with meal) (9)

SNACK—Banana-Almond Yogurt (266)
Banana-Almond Yogurt
8 ounces sugar-free, nonfat yogurt (98)
1 small banana (90)
2 tablespoons slivered almonds (78)

DAY 21 Nutritional Values
Calories—2,011
Fiber (g)—26.52
GI = all<70
% Fat—38.31
% SFA—6.74
% MUFA—16.36
% PUFA—13.14
AA (mg)—140
EPA (mg)—510
Cholesterol (mg)—187

* You'll find recipes for items marked with an asterisk * in chapter 18.

DAY 22

BREAKFAST—Pancakes with Margarine and Peaches, Milk
3 (4-inch) whole-wheat pancakes prepared from mix with liquid egg substitute (275)
2 teaspoons trans-fat-free margarine (58)
1 cup peaches (59)
1 cup 1% milk (102)

1 borage oil capsule (taken with meal) (9)

LUNCH—Roast Beef Pita (417), Asparagus Salad (150)
Roast Beef Pita
3-ounces cooked lean eye of round beef (143)
1 (6-inch) whole-wheat pita (170)
1 tablespoon no-cholesterol mayonnaise (103)
1 leaf lettuce (1)

Asparagus Salad
¾ cup cooked asparagus (30)
1 tablespoon canola oil (120)
Vinegar, lemon juice, and herbs of choice

DINNER—Pork Tenderloin Stir-Fry (366), Brown Rice, Roll with Margarine, Vanilla Pudding with Strawberries
Pork Tenderloin Stir-Fry
4 ounces pork tenderloin (186)
½ cup sliced green peppers (9)
½ cup sliced red peppers (12)
½ cup chopped broccoli (7)
½ cup sliced mushrooms (8)
½ cup sliced onions (24)
1 tablespoon canola oil to stir-fry pork and vegetables (120)

1 cup cooked brown rice (216)
1 small whole-wheat roll (75)
1 teaspoon trans-fat-free margarine (29)
½ cup sugar-free, nonfat vanilla pudding (75)
1 cup strawberries (53)

1 borage oil capsule (taken with meal) (9)

SNACK—Celery Stuffed with Pimento Cheese
2 stalks celery (11)
1 ounce processed pimento cheese spread (106)

DAY 22 Nutritional Values
Calories—2,010
Fiber (g)—28.15
GI = all<70
% Fat—38.38
% SFA—8.95
% MUFA—15.54
% PUFA—11.40
AA (mg)—80
EPA (mg)—0
Cholesterol (mg)—268

DAY 23

BREAKFAST—Cheese Toast (264), Citrus Sections
Cheese Toast
2 slices multigrain bread (130)
2 teaspoons trans-fat-free margarine, 70% vegetable oil spread (58)
1½ ounces low-fat cheese (76)

¾ cup orange sections (63)
¾ cup grapefruit sections (55)

1 borage oil capsule (taken with meal) (9)

LUNCH—Ham⸏nd-Broccoli Pasta Salad (561), Bran Muⁱⁿ
Ham-and-Broccoli Pasta Salad
3 ounces lean cooked ham (123)
2 ounces part-skim mozzarella cheese (171)
1 cup cooked spiral shaped macaroni (189)
½ cup chopped fresh broccoli (15)
6 cherry tomatoes, halved (18)
¼ cup low-fat Italian dressing (45)

1 medium low-fat muffin (169)

DINNER—Scalloped Oysters* (392), Spinach Salad with Vinaigrette Dressing (91), Roll with Margarine, Apple
Scalloped Oysters
5 ounces eastern oysters (112)
¼ cup plain bread crumbs (107)
2 tablespoons trans-fat-free margarine (173)

Spinach Salad with Vinaigrette Dressing
1 cup fresh spinach (7)
¼ cup sliced mushrooms (4)
2 teaspoons olive oil (80)
Raspberry vinegar and herbs of choice

1 small oat-bran dinner roll (67)
1 teaspoon trans-fat-free margarine (29)
½ cup cooked apples (73)

1 borage oil capsule (taken with meal) (9)

SNACK—Sugar-Free, Nonfat Frozen Yogurt with Peaches
1 cup sugar-free nonfat frozen yogurt (199)
1 small peach (31)

DAY 23 Nutritional Values
Calories—2,012
Fiber (g)—24.82
GI = all<70
% Fat—35.70
% SFA—10.08
% MUFA—15.68
% PUFA—7.54
AA (mg)—70
EPA (mg)—320
Cholesterol (mg)—178

* You'll find recipes for items marked with an asterisk * in chapter 18.

DAY 24

BREAKFAST—Oatmeal with Apricots and Milk, Apple Juice
1 cup cooked oatmeal (145)
⅓ cup dried apricots (103)
1 cup 1% milk (102)
4 ounces unsweetened apple juice (58)

1 borage oil capsule (taken with meal) (9)

LUNCH—Curried Shrimp Salad* (706), Crackers, Waldorf-Gelatin Salad (121)
Curried Shrimp Salad
5 ounces cooked shrimp (140)
1 cup cooked brown rice (216)
⅓ cup cooked green peas (41)
3 tablespoons no-cholesterol
    mayonnaise (309)

6 whole-wheat crackers (106)

Sugar-Free Waldorf-Gelatin Salad
½ cup sugar-free prepared gelatin (9)
¼ cup diced apples (14)
2 tablespoons chopped English walnuts (98)

DINNER—Sirloin Steak Roquefort (376), Sweet Potato, Green Beans
Sirloin Steak Roquefort
5 ounces lean beef top sirloin (276), broiled
    or grilled with 1 ounce blue cheese (100)

1 medium baked sweet potato (103)
1 cup cooked green beans (38)
1 teaspoon trans-fat-free margarine (29)

1 borage oil capsule (taken with meal) (9)

SNACK—Whole-Wheat Pretzels
1 ounce whole-wheat pretzels (103)

DAY 24 Nutritional Values
Calories—2,008
Fiber (g)—29.32
GI = all<70
% Fat—36.19
% SFA—9.00
% MUFA—10.10
% PUFA—15.39
AA (mg)—160
EPA (mg)—240
Cholesterol (mg)—436

---

* You'll find recipes for items marked with an asterisk * in chapter 18.

DAY 25

BREAKFAST—MultiGrain Cheerios with Milk and Banana, Mozzarella Cheese Stick
¾ cup MultiGrain Cheerios cereal (81)
1 cup 1% milk (102)
1 small banana (90)
1 ounce part-skim mozzarella
   cheese stick (86)

1 borage oil capsule (taken with meal) (9)

LUNCH—Barbeque Beef Pita Pizza (308), Corn-and-Black-Bean Salad (255)
Barbeque Beef Pita Pizza
1 (4-inch) whole-wheat pita
   (for pizza crust) (74)
2 tablespoons barbeque sauce (23)
3 ounces cooked ground beef
   (95% lean) (145)
¼ cup chopped onion (17)
1 ounce low-fat cheese (49)

Corn-and-Black-Bean Salad
¼ cup yellow corn (151)
¼ cup canned black beans (55)
2 tablespoons chopped green pepper (4)
2 tablespoons chopped red pepper (5)
1 teaspoon canola oil (40)
Vinegar, lemon juice, cilantro,
   and spices of choice

DINNER—Oven-Fried Chicken (249), Carrots, Tossed Salad with Ranch Dressing, Baked Apple Crisp (224)
Oven-Fried Chicken
4 ounces cooked chicken breast
   (no skin) (196)
2 tablespoons plain bread crumbs (53)

1 cup cooked carrots (55)
2 tablespoons trans-fat-free margarine (173)

Tossed Salad with Low-Fat
Ranch Dressing
1 cup lettuce (6)
¼ cup sliced cucumber (4)
¼ cup grated carrots (11)
2 tablespoons low-fat ranch dressing (68)

Baked Apple Crisp
1 cup apple slices (53)
2 tablespoons oats (76)
2 tablespoons sliced almonds (66)
1 teaspoon trans-fat-free margarine (29)

1 borage oil capsule (taken with meal) (9)

SNACK—Ham-and-Cheese Pinwheels (277)
Ham-and-Cheese Pinwheels
1 (6-inch) flour tortilla (150)
1 ounce extra lean ham (37)
2 tablespoons low-fat cream cheese (69)
1 tablespoon diced green pepper (2)
2 tablespoons diced black olives (19)

DAY 25 Nutritional Values
Calories—2,007
Fiber (g)—29.58
GI = all<70
% Fat—35.38
% SFA—10.18
% MUFA—15.69
% PUFA—6.93
AA (mg)—130
EPA (mg)—10
Cholesterol (mg)—231

DAY 26

BREAKFAST—Bran Muffin with Margarine, Fruit Salad
2 ounces low-fat bran muffin (153)
1 teaspoon trans-fat-free margarine (29)

Fruit Salad
¼ cup kiwi (27)
¼ cup pineapple (19)
¼ cup blueberries (21)
¼ cup peaches (17)

1 borage oil capsule (taken with meal) (9)

LUNCH—Philly Cheese Steak Sandwich (519), Vinaigrette Coleslaw (112), Fresh Peach
Philly Cheese Steak Sandwich
1 whole-wheat hoagie roll (173)
3 ounces cooked lean beef tenderloin (179)
¾ cup sliced onions (36)
½ teaspoon canola oil to sauté beef and onions (20)
1 ounce provolone cheese (100)
1 tablespoon Worcestershire sauce (11)

Vinaigrette Coleslaw
1½ cups chopped cabbage (32)
2 teaspoons canola oil (80)
Vinegar, sugar substitute, and spices of choice

1 small peach (31)

DINNER—Salmon in Sun-Dried-Tomato Cream Sauce with Pasta* (749), Wilted Spinach with Pine Nuts (87)
Salmon in Sun-Dried-Tomato Cream Sauce
4 ounces cooked or canned wild salmon (or other Category 1 fish) (245)
½ cup white sauce (184)
1 ounce grated fresh Parmesan cheese (111)
¼ cup sun-dried tomatoes (35)
1 cup whole-wheat pasta (174)

Wilted Spinach with Pine Nuts
1 cup spinach (40) cooked with 1 teaspoon olive oil (41)
10 dried pine nuts (6)

1 borage oil capsule (taken with meal) (9)

SNACK—Yogurt with Blueberries and Almonds
Yogurt with Blueberries and Almonds
8 ounces sugar-free nonfat yogurt (98)
¾ cup blueberries (62)
2 tablespoons sliced almonds (66)

DAY 26 Nutritional Values
Calories—2,008
Fiber (g)—30.73
GI = all<70
% Fat—37.50
% SFA—10.33
% MUFA—16.45
% PUFA—8.32
AA (mg)—70
EPA (mg)—600
Cholesterol (mg)—222

* You'll find recipes for items marked with an asterisk * in chapter 18.

DAY 27

BREAKFAST—Scrambled Egg Substitute, Toast with Margarine and Jelly, Canadian Bacon, Grapefruit
½ cup cooked liquid egg substitute (105)
1 ounce Canadian-style bacon (45)
2 slices whole-wheat bread (138)
2 teaspoons trans-fat-free margarine (58)
2 tablespoons reduced- or no-sugar
   jelly (68)
½ medium grapefruit (41)

1 borage oil capsule (taken with meal) (9)

LUNCH—Oriental Grilled Chicken Salad with Citrus Vinaigrette (496), Sliced Tomatoes
Oriental Grilled Chicken Salad
  with Citrus Vinaigrette
2 cups green leaf lettuce (17)
4 ounces cooked chicken breast
  (no skin) (196)
¼ cup grated carrot (11)
¼ cup chopped green onions (8)
¼ cup mandarin oranges (23)
2 tablespoons Chinese chow mein
  noodles (30)
2 tablespoons slivered almonds (78)
1 tablespoon canola oil (120)
1 ounce unsweetened orange juice (13)

1 large tomato (33)

DINNER—Pecan-Crusted Pork Chop (348), Asparagus, Wild Rice, Poached Pear
Pecan-Crusted Pork Chop
4 ounces cooked lean top loin pork
  chop (194)
2 tablespoons minced pecans (94)
½ tablespoon canola oil (60)

1 cup cooked asparagus (40)
1 cup cooked wild rice (166)
1 medium pear (96)

1 borage oil capsule (taken with meal) (9)

SNACK—Trail Mix (354)
Trail Mix
¼ cup slivered almonds (156)
6 dried apricot halves (51)
6 dried apple rings (93)
2 tablespoons Grape-Nuts (54)

DAY 27 Nutritional Values
Calories—2,006
Fiber (g)—35.38
GI = all<70
% Fat—35.82
% SFA—5.11
% MUFA—18.71
% PUFA—10.22
AA (mg)—160
EPA (mg)—10
Cholesterol (mg)—197

DAY 28

BREAKFAST—Bagel with Cream Cheese, Tomato and Lox, Cranapple Juice
1 small oat-bran bagel (66)
2 ounces lox (Chinook smoked salmon) (66)
2 tablespoons low-fat cream cheese (69)
2 slices fresh tomato (7)
6 ounces low-calorie cranapple juice (34)

1 borage oil capsule (taken with meal) (9)

LUNCH—Cheeseburger, Baked Beans, Dill Pickle, Apple
Cheeseburger
1 whole-wheat hamburger roll (114)
4 ounces cooked ground beef
    (95% lean) (194)
¾ ounce low-fat cheese (38)
1 tablespoon no-cholesterol mayonnaise
    (103)

1 large dill pickle (24)
¾ cup vegetarian baked beans (177)
1 small apple (55)

DINNER—Grilled Shrimp* (220), Orange Rice Bake (267), Green Beans, Strawberries and Bananas
Grilled Shrimp
5 ounces cooked shrimp (140)
2 teaspoons canola oil (80)

Orange Rice Bake
1 cup cooked brown rice (215)
4 ounces unsweetened orange juice (used as
    part of liquid for cooking rice) (52)

1 cup cooked green beans (38)
1 tablespoon trans-fat-free margarine (87)
¾ cup strawberries (40)
¾ cup sliced bananas (100)

1 borage oil capsule (taken with meal) (9)

SNACK—Dry-Roasted Peanuts
⅓ cup dry-roasted peanuts (282)

DAY 28 Nutritional Values
Calories—1,999
Fiber (g)—35.59
GI = all<70
% Fat—35.17
% SFA—7.93
% MUFA—14.92
% PUFA—10.97
AA (mg)—160
EPA (mg)—350
Cholesterol (mg)—400

* You'll find recipes for items marked with an asterisk * in chapter 18.

Chapter Seventeen
The Chilton Solution Diet

The Chilton Solution Prescription

For people living with inflammatory disease.

- Eat foods whose values add up to no more than 100 on the Inflammatory Index per day.

- Eat an average of at least 400 milligrams a day of EPA. This equates to roughly four servings of Category 1 or 2 fish a week, or five servings of Category 3 fish. If you'd prefer to supplement instead, take one capsule (typically 150 to 180 milligrams) of EPA three times daily, with breakfast, lunch, and dinner.

- Take an average of at least 650 to 950 milligrams of GLA a day in supplement form, which means a capsule (typically about 210 to 240 milligrams) three times daily, with breakfast, lunch, and dinner.

- DO NOT take the recommended doses of GLA without having EPA—either through the fish you're eating or by supplementation in your diet.

- Choose carbohydrates with a low-to-moderate Glycemic Index value.

DAY 1

BREAKFAST—Scrambled Egg Substitute, English Muffin with Margarine and Jelly, Tomato Juice
½ cup cooked liquid egg substitute (105)
1 whole-wheat English muffin (134)
2 teaspoons trans-fat-free margarine (58)
2 tablespoons reduced- or no-sugar jelly
    (68)
6 ounces tomato juice (31)

1 borage oil capsule (taken with meal) (9)

LUNCH—Cheeseburger on Bun (307), Tossed Salad with Vinaigrette, Fresh Apple
Cheeseburger on Bun
1 multigrain hamburger bun (113)
3 ounces cooked ground beef
    (95% lean) (145)
1 ounce low-fat cheese (49)

Tossed Salad with Vinaigrette Dressing
1 cup green leaf lettuce (8)
¼ cup sliced cucumbers (4)
4 cherry tomatoes (12)
1 tablespoon vinegar and oil salad
    dressing (72)
1 medium apple (72)

1 borage oil capsule (taken with meal) (9)

DINNER—Lemon-Herb Mackerel* (297), Brown Rice Pilaf (349), Broccoli Parmesan (155), Roll with Margarine
4 ounces broiled or grilled Atlantic mackerel
    (or another Category 1 fish) (297)

Brown Rice Pilaf
1 cup cooked brown rice (216)
¼ cup cooked grated carrots (14)
1 tablespoon olive oil (119)

Broccoli Parmesan
1 cup cooked broccoli (44)
1 ounce grated fresh Parmesan cheese (111)

1 small whole-wheat dinner roll (75)
½ tablespoon trans-fat-free margarine (43)

1 borage oil capsule (taken with meal) (9)

SNACK—Peach Smoothe (189)
Peach Smoothie
½ cup 1% milk (51)
½ cup sugar-free, nonfat frozen yogurt (100)
1 medium peach (38)

DAY 1 Nutritional Values
Calories—2,006
Fiber (g)—27.33
GI = all<70
% Fat—37.65
% SFA—10.30
% MUFA—16.56
% PUFA—8.45
AA (mg)—100
EPA (mg)—570
Cholesterol (mg)—186

* You'll find recipes for items marked with an asterisk * in chapter 18.

Note. See explanation of nutritional value abbreviations on page 177.

DAY 2

BREAKFAST—Grapefruit, Omelet (185), Toast with Margarine and Jelly
½ medium grapefruit (41)

Omelet
½ cup cooked liquid egg substitute (105)
¼ cup chopped green peppers (8)
½ ounce diced Canadian bacon (23)
1 ounce grated low-fat cheese (49)

2 slices oat-bran bread (142)
2 teaspoons trans-fat-free margarine (58)
1 tablespoon reduced- or no-sugar jelly (34)

1 borage oil capsule (taken with meal) (9)

LUNCH—Waldorf Tuna Salad* (471), Crackers, Carrot and Pepper Strips, Pudding with Strawberries
Waldorf Tuna Salad
4 ounces canned white tuna (145)
2 tablespoons no-cholesterol
   mayonnaise (206)
¼ cup chopped apple (14)
¼ cup chopped celery (4)
2 tablespoons chopped English
   walnuts (102)

½ cup carrot strips (25)
½ cup red pepper strips (12)
8 whole-wheat crackers (142)
½ cup sugar-free, nonfat vanilla
   pudding (75)
1 cup strawberries (53)

1 borage oil capsule (taken with meal) (9)

DINNER—Barbeque Pork Chop, Yellow Corn, Asparagus, Cucumber-Tomato Salad (96), Roll with Margarine
4 ounces lean top loin pork chop (194)
   cooked with 1 tablespoon barbeque
   sauce (12)
1 cup cooked asparagus (40)
1 cup cooked yellow corn (177)

Cucumber-Tomato Salad
⅓ cup sliced cucumbers (5)
⅓ cup chopped tomato (11)
2 teaspoons olive oil (80)
Vinegar and herbs of choice

1 small whole-wheat dinner roll (75)
1 tablespoon trans-fat-free margarine (29)

1 borage oil capsule (taken with meal) (9)

SNACK—Yogurt Crunch (128)
Yogurt Crunch
8 ounces sugar-free, nonfat yogurt (98)
¼ cup Fiber One cereal (30)

DAY 2 Nutritional Values
Calories—2,016
Fiber (g)—35.03
GI = all<70
% Fat—38.76
% SFA—6.96
% MUFA—14.0
% PUFA—15.36
AA (mg)—90
EPA (mg)—260
Cholesterol (mg)—152

* You'll find recipes for items marked with an asterisk * in chapter 18.

DAY 3

BREAKFAST—Cottage Cheese with Berries, Oat-Bran Muffin with Margarine
½ cup 1% cottage cheese (81)
½ cup blueberries (41)
½ cup strawberries (27)
1 medium low-fat oat-bran muffin (305)
1 teaspoon trans-fat-free margarine (29)

1 borage oil capsule (taken with meal) (9)

LUNCH—Oriental Flank Steak Salad with Orange Vinaigrette (353), Roll, Fruit Salad (91)
Oriental Flank Steak Salad with
Orange Vinaigrette
2 cups green leaf lettuce (17)
3 ounces cooked beef flank steak (158)
¼ cup mandarin oranges (23)
¼ cup grated carrots (11)
¼ cup sliced red onions (12)
1 tablespoon peanut oil (119)
1 ounce unsweetened orange juice (13)
Vinegar and spices of choice

1 small whole-wheat dinner roll (75)

Fruit Salad
⅓ cup kiwi (36)
⅓ cup grapes (37)
⅓ cup strawberries (18)

1 borage oil capsule (taken with meal) (9)

DINNER—Broiled Salmon* (367), Green Beans Almandine (203), Baked Sweet Potato, Baked Apple
6 ounces cooked wild sockeye salmon (or another Category 1 fish) (367)

Green Beans Almandine
1 cup cooked green beans (38)
2 tablespoons slivered almonds (78)
1 tablespoon trans-fat-free margarine (87)

1 medium baked sweet potato (103)
1 medium apple, baked with cinnamon (72)

1 borage oil capsule (taken with meal) (9)

SNACK—Crackers with Cheese
8 whole-wheat crackers (142)
2 ounces low-fat cheese (98)

DAY 3 Nutritional Values	
Calories—2,014	
Fiber (g)—31.24	
GI = all<70	
% Fat—35.89	
% SFA—7.77	
% MUFA—15.95	
% PUFA—9.36	
AA (mg)—80	
EPA (mg)—900	
Cholesterol (mg)—206	

* You'll find recipes for items marked with an asterisk * in chapter 18.

DAY 4

BREAKFAST—Cranapple Juice, Loaded Muffin (349)

6 ounces low-calorie cranapple juice (34)

Loaded Muffin
1 multigrain English muffin (155)
2 teaspoons trans-fat-free margarine (58)
¼ cup cooked liquid egg substitute (53)
1 ounce Canadian bacon (45)
¾ ounce low-fat American cheese (38)

1 borage oil capsule (taken with meal) (9)

LUNCH—Beef-and-Provolone Pita (441), Spinach Salad with Vinaigrette Dressing (167), Fresh Peach

Beef-and-Provolone Pita
1 (6-inch) whole-wheat pita (170)
2 tablespoons low-fat ranch salad
    dressing (66)
2 ounces cooked lean eye of round beef (95)
1 ounce provolone cheese (100)
1 leaf lettuce (2)
¼ cup chopped tomatoes (8)

Spinach Salad with Vinaigrette Dressing
1 cup fresh spinach (7)
1 slice lean cooked bacon (37)
¼ cup sliced mushrooms (4)
1 tablespoon olive oil (119)
Vinegar and herbs of choice

1 small peach (31)

1 borage oil capsule (taken with meal) (9)

DINNER—Grilled Pork Tenderloin Dijon, Lemon Couscous, Snow Peas, Frozen Yogurt

Grilled Pork Tenderloin Dijon
4 ounces cooked pork tenderloin (186)
1 teaspoon Dijon mustard (for basting) (3)

Lemon Couscous
1 cup couscous, cooked with lemon juice
    and lemon zest added (176)

1 cup cooked snow peas (83)
1 tablespoon trans-fat-free margarine (87)
1 cup sugar-free, nonfat frozen yogurt (199)

1 borage oil capsule (taken with meal) (9)

SNACK—MultiGrain Cheerios with Milk and Blackberries

1 cup MultiGrain Cheerios (108)
¾ cup 1% milk (77)
½ cup blueberries (41)

DAY 4 Nutritional Values
Calories—2,009
Fiber (g)—25.24
GI = all<70
% Fat—31.58
% SFA—8.78
% MUFA—14.48
% PUFA—5.04
AA (mg)—60
EPA (mg)—0
Cholesterol (mg)—202

DAY 5

BREAKFAST—Whole-Wheat Pancakes (403), Canadian Bacon, Apple Slices
Whole-Wheat Pancakes
½ cup whole-wheat pancake mix (241)
½ cup 1% milk (51)
¼ cup cooked liquid egg substitute (53)
2 teaspoons trans-fat-free margarine (58)

1 cup apple slices (97)
1 ounce Canadian bacon (45)

1 borage oil capsule (taken with meal) (9)

LUNCH—Chicken Salad (254), Crackers, Marinated Cucumbers (48), Strawberries
Chicken Salad
3 ounces cooked chicken breast
   (no skin) (147)
1 tablespoon no-cholesterol
   mayonnaise (103)
¼ cup chopped celery (4)

8 whole-wheat crackers (142)

Marinated Cucumbers
½ cup sliced cucumbers (8)
1 teaspoon canola oil (40)
Vinegar, herbs, and spices of choice

1 cup strawberries (53)

1 borage oil capsule (taken with meal) (9)

DINNER—Crab Cakes* (538), Broccoli, Broiled Tomato, Dinner Roll with Margarine
Crab Cakes
6 ounces Alaskan-king-crab meat (165)
2 tablespoons cooked liquid egg
   substitute (26)
¼ cup plain bread crumbs (107)
2 tablespoons canola oil to fry crab
   cakes (240)

1 large tomato (33)
1 cup cooked broccoli (44)
1 small whole-wheat roll (75)
1 teaspoon trans-fat-free margarine (29)

1 borage oil capsule (taken with meal) (9)

SNACK—Yogurt-Banana Split (227)
Yogurt-Banana Split
8 ounces sugar-free, nonfat yogurt (98)
1 small banana (90)
1 tablespoon slivered almonds (39)

DAY 5 Nutritional Values
Calories—2,015
Fiber (g)—25.40
GI = all<70
% Fat—36.72
% SFA—5.47
% MUFA—15.67
% PUFA—13.0
AA (mg)—140
EPA (mg)—510
Cholesterol (mg)—188

* You'll find recipes for items marked with an asterisk * in chapter 18.

DAY 6

BREAKFAST—Bagel with Cream Cheese, Grapefruit

1 medium oat-bran bagel (181)
2 tablespoons low-fat cream cheese (69)
½ medium grapefruit (41)

1 borage oil capsule (taken with meal) (9)

LUNCH—Hawaiian Pizza Salad with Vinaigrette Dressing (360), Crackers, Grapes

Hawaiian Pizza Salad with Vinaigrette Dressing
2 cups green leaf lettuce (17)
2 ounces part-skim mozzarella cheese (144)
2 ounces lean ham (92)
¼ cup pineapple (19)
½ cup chopped tomato (16)
1 tablespoon vinegar and oil salad
    dressing (72)

5 whole-wheat crackers (89)

2 cups grapes (221)

1 borage oil capsule (taken with meal) (9)

DINNER—Shrimp Cocktail, Beef Tenderloin Roquefort (289), Zucchini au Gratin (168), Baked Sweet Potato, Poached Pears

4 ounces cooked shrimp (112)
2 tablespoons seafood cocktail sauce (35)

Beef Tenderloin Roquefort
4 ounces broiled or grilled lean beef
    tenderloin (239) with ½ ounce blue
    cheese (50)

1 medium baked sweet potato (103)
1 teaspoon trans-fat-free margarine (29)

Zucchini au Gratin
1 cup cooked zucchini (29)
1 teaspoon olive oil (40)
1 tablespoon plain bread crumbs (27)
1 ounce part-skim mozzarella cheese (72)

¾ cup pears (53)

1 borage oil capsule (taken with meal) (9)

SNACK—Pistachios
⅓ cup dry-roasted pistachios (231)

DAY 6 Nutritional Values
Calories—2,008
Fiber (g)—28.46
GI = all<70
% Fat—36.55
% SFA—12.33
% MUFA—14.73
% PUFA—6.95
AA (mg)—150
EPA (mg)—190
Cholesterol (mg)—431

DAY 7

BREAKFAST—Oatmeal with Blueberries (186), Cheese Toast, Apple Juice
1 cup cooked oatmeal (145)
½ cup blueberries (41)

Cheese Toast
1 slice whole-wheat bread (69)
1 teaspoon trans-fat-free margarine (29)
1 ounce low-fat cheese (51)

4 ounces unsweetened apple juice (58)

1 borage oil capsule (taken with meal) (9)

LUNCH—Roasted Pork Sandwich (348), Coleslaw (133), Cantaloupe
Roasted Pork Sandwich
1 whole-wheat hamburger roll (114)
3 ounces cooked lean top loin pork
  roast (165)
2 teaspoons no-cholesterol mayonnaise (69)

Coleslaw
1 cup chopped cabbage (21)
2 tablespoons reduced fat coleslaw
  dressing (112)

2 cups cantaloupe (109)

1 borage oil capsule (taken with meal) (9)

DINNER—Lemon-Herb Salmon* (306), Lentils au Gratin (313), Caesar Salad
5 ounces broiled or grilled sockeye salmon
  (or another Category 1 fish) (306)

Lentils au Gratin
1 cup cooked lentils (230)
1 tablespoon plain bread crumbs (27)
½ ounce grated fresh Parmesan cheese (56)

Caesar Salad
1 cup romaine lettuce (10)
2 tablespoons plain croutons (15)
2 tablespoons low-fat Caesar salad
  dressing (33)
½ ounce grated fresh Parmesan cheese (56)

1 borage oil capsule (taken with meal) (9)

SNACK—Apple with Peanut Butter
1 medium apple (72)
2 tablespoons peanut butter (192)

DAY 7 Nutritional Values
Calories—2,007
Fiber (g)—38.6
GI = all<70
% Fat—34.20
% SFA—8.50
% MUFA—13.91
% PUFA—8.47
AA (mg)—70
EPA (mg)—750
Cholesterol (mg)—228

* You'll find recipes for items marked with an asterisk * in chapter 18.

DAY 8

**BREAKFAST—Granola (374)
with Berries and Milk**
Granola
¼ cup oats (152)
1 tablespoon honey (64)
1 tablespoon toasted sunflower seeds (50)
2 tablespoons chopped English
   walnuts (102)
2 tablespoons low-calorie cranapple juice (6)

¼ cup strawberries (13)
¼ cup raspberries (16)
¼ cup blueberries (21)
1 cup 1% milk (102)

1 borage oil capsule (taken with meal) (9)

LUNCH—Steak Sandwich (374), Grapes
Steak Sandwich
1 multigrain hamburger roll (113)
3 ounces cooked beef flank steak (158)
1 tablespoon no-cholesterol
   mayonnaise (103)

1 cup grapes (110)

1 borage oil capsule (taken with meal) (9)

**DINNER—Italian Chicken (478), Spaghetti,
Green Beans Vinaigrette (74),
Tossed Salad with Italian Dressing (41)**
Italian Chicken
4 ounces cooked chicken breast (no skin)
   (196)
2 tablespoons seasoned bread crumbs (55)
1 tablespoon olive oil to cook chicken (119)
¼ cup marinara sauce (36)
1 ounce part-skim mozzarella cheese (72)

1 cup cooked whole-wheat spaghetti (174)

Green Beans Vinaigrette
1 cup cooked green beans (38)
1 tablespoon diced sweet red peppers (2)
1 tablespoon reduced- or no-sugar jelly (34)
Vinegar and spices of choice

Tossed Salad with Italian Dressing
1 cup romaine lettuce (10)
3 cherry tomatoes (9)
2 tablespoons low-fat Italian dressing (22)

1 borage oil capsule (taken with meal) (9)

SNACK—Ricotta Apple Pie (198)
Ricotta Apple Pie
½ cup low-fat ricotta cheese (170)
½ small apple, diced (28)
1 teaspoon cinnamon and spices

DAY 8 Nutritional Values
Calories—2,002
Fiber (g)—28.68
GI = all<70
% Fat—35.80
% SFA—9.76
% MUFA—12.67
% PUFA—10.96
AA (mg)—120
EPA (mg)—10
Cholesterol (mg)—208

DAY 9

BREAKFAST—Veggie-and-Ricotta Frittata (207), Toast with Margarine and Jelly, Tomato Juice
Veggie-and-Ricotta Frittata
½ cup cooked liquid egg substitute (105)
2 tablespoons low-fat ricotta cheese (42)
¼ cup sliced summer squash (5)
¼ cup chopped sweet red peppers (10)
1 ounce diced Canadian bacon (45)

1 slice multigrain bread (65)
1 teaspoon trans-fat-free margarine (29)
1 tablespoon reduced- or no-sugar jelly (34)
8 ounces tomato juice (41)

1 borage oil capsule (taken with meal) (9)

LUNCH—Grilled Tuna Salad* with Ranch Dressing (313), Three-Bean Salad (205), Crackers
Grilled Tuna Salad with Low-Fat
Ranch Dressing
2 cups red leaf lettuce (9)
4 ounces grilled or broiled wild bluefin
    tuna (209)
¼ cup chopped onion (17)
¼ cup grated carrots (11)
2 tablespoons low-fat ranch salad
    dressing (67)

Three-Bean Salad
¼ cup canned green beans (7)
¼ cup canned chickpeas (71)
¼ cup canned wax beans (7)
1 tablespoon canola oil (120)
Vinegar, herbs, and spices of choice

5 whole-wheat crackers (87)

1 borage oil capsule (taken with meal) (9)

DINNER—Italian Pork Chops (212), Baked Brown Rice (253), Sautéed Spinach with Pine Nuts (179), Apple
Italian Pork Chops
3 ounces cooked lean pork loin chops (145)
¼ cup sliced green pepper (5)
½ medium onion (23)
½ cup tomato sauce (39)

Baked Brown Rice
1 cup cooked brown rice (216)
2 tablespoons condensed beef broth
    (used in cooking rice) (8)
1 teaspoon trans-fat-free margarine (29)

Sautéed Spinach with Pine Nuts
1 cup spinach (41), sautéed with
    1 tablespoon olive oil (119)
30 dried pine nuts (19)

1 medium apple (72)

1 borage oil capsule (taken with meal) (9)

SNACK—Peach Yogurt Crunch (272)
Peach Yogurt Crunch
1 cup sugar-free, nonfat yogurt (98)
1 medium peach (38)
2 tablespoons oats (76)
2 tablespoons sliced almonds (60)

DAY 9 Nutritional Values
Calories—1,996
Fiber (g)—31.21
GI = all<70
% Fat—34.75
% SFA—6.01
% MUFA—15.90
% PUFA—9.58
AA (mg)—110
EPA (mg)—410
Cholesterol (mg)—155

* You'll find recipes for items marked with an asterisk * in chapter 18.

DAY 10

BREAKFAST—Western Omelet Wrap (389), Grapefruit

Western Omelet Wrap

1 (10-inch) flour tortilla (227)
½ cup cooked liquid egg substitute (105)
1 ounce diced Canadian-style bacon (45)
2 tablespoons chopped green pepper (4)
2 tablespoons chopped onion (8)

½ medium grapefruit (41)

1 borage oil capsule (taken with meal) (9)

LUNCH—Greek Salmon Salad* (502), Whole-Wheat Pita, Strawberries and Yogurt

Greek Salmon Salad

2 cups romaine lettuce (19)
4 ounces cooked or canned wild salmon (or another Category 1 fish) (245)
½ cup chopped tomatoes (16)
2 tablespoons chopped green onions (4)
¼ cup sliced cucumbers (4)
1 ounce feta cheese (75)
4 large ripe black olives (20)
1 tablespoon olive oil (119)
Vinegar and herbs of choice

1 (4-inch) whole-wheat pita (74)
1 cup strawberries (53)
8 ounces sugar-free, nonfat yogurt (98)

1 borage oil capsule (taken with meal) (9)

DINNER—Roast Beef, Roasted Vegetables (191), Baked Sweet Potato, Roll with Margarine

4 ounces cooked lean eye of round beef (191)
1 medium baked sweet potato (103)
1 teaspoon trans-fat-free margarine (29)

Roasted Vegetables

1 cup sliced summer squash (18)
6 asparagus spears (19)
¼ chopped medium onion (12)
¼ cup chopped eggplant (5)
6 cherry tomatoes (18)
1 tablespoon olive oil (119)

1 small whole-wheat dinner roll (75)
1 teaspoon trans-fat-free margarine (29)

1 borage oil capsule (taken with meal) (9)

SNACK—Chocolate-Banana Pudding

¾ cup sugar-free, nonfat chocolate pudding (111)
1 small banana (90)

DAY 10 Nutritional Values
Calories—2,003
Fiber (g)—28.37
GI = all<70
% Fat—35.20
% SFA—7.93
% MUFA—18.37
% PUFA—5.72
AA (mg)—60
EPA (mg)—600
Cholesterol (mg)—222

* You'll find recipes for items marked with an asterisk* in chapter 18.

DAY 11

BREAKFAST—Yogurt, Bagel with Cream Cheese, Cantaloupe
6 ounces sugar-free, nonfat yogurt (73)
½ medium oat-bran bagel (73)
2 tablespoons low-fat cream cheese (69)
1 cup cantaloupe (54)

1 borage oil capsule (taken with meal) (9)

LUNCH—Chicken Quesadilla (622), Tomato Salad (157), Fresh Apple
Chicken Quesadilla
1 (10-inch) flour tortilla (227)
2 ounces cooked chicken breast
    (no skin) (98)
¼ sliced small onion (12)
¼ cup sliced green peppers (4)
¼ cup sliced red peppers (5)
1 tablespoon canola oil to sauté chicken
    and vegetables (120)
2 ounces low-fat cheese (98)
2 tablespoons low-fat sour cream (40)
¼ cup salsa (18)

Tomato Salad
½ cup halved cherry tomatoes (13)
2 tablespoons vinegar-and-oil salad
    dressing (144)

1 small apple (55)

1 borage oil capsule (taken with meal) (9)

DINNER—Shrimp-and-Vegetable Stir-Fry II* (505), Roll with Margarine
Shrimp-and-Vegetable Stir-Fry II
3 ounces cooked shrimp (84)
½ cup snow peas (42)
½ cup sliced red onions (34)
1 cup halved cherry tomatoes (32)
½ cup sliced red bell peppers (19)
1 tablespoon olive oil to sauté shrimp and
    vegetables (120)

1 cup cooked whole-wheat spaghetti (174)

1 medium whole-wheat dinner roll (96)
1 teaspoon trans-fat-free margarine (29)

1 borage oil capsule (taken with meal) (9)

SNACK—Crackers with Tuna Salad* (180)
4 whole-wheat crackers (71)

Tuna Salad
3 ounces canned white tuna (109)
2 teaspoons no-cholesterol mayonnaise (69)
2 tablespoons chopped celery (2)

DAY 11 Nutritional Values
Calories—2,011
Fiber (g)—28.49
GI = all<70
% Fat—38.73
% SFA—8.81
% MUFA—15.21
% PUFA—12.90
AA (mg)—150
EPA (mg)—350
Cholesterol (mg)—294

* You'll find recipes for items marked with an asterisk* in chapter 18.

DAY 12

BREAKFAST—Scrambled Egg Substitute, Canadian Bacon, Toast with Margarine and Jelly, Citrus Sections

½ cup cooked liquid egg substitute (105)
2 ounces Canadian style bacon (89)
2 slices oat-bran bread (142)
2 teaspoons trans-fat-free margarine (58)
2 tablespoons reduced- or no-sugar jelly (68)
¾ cup orange sections (61)
¾ cup grapefruit sections (55)

1 borage oil capsule (taken with meal) (9)

LUNCH—Portabella-and-Provolone Sandwich (375), Mixed-Cabbage-and-Apple Salad (79), Strawberry Smoothie (151)

Portabella-and-Provolone Sandwich
1 multigrain hamburger roll (147)
3 ounces grilled portabella mushroom (22)
1 ounce provolone cheese (100)
1 tablespoon no-cholesterol mayonnaise dressing (103)
2 leaves green leaf lettuce (3)

Mixed-Cabbage-and-Apple Salad
¼ cup shredded Chinese cabbage (2)
¼ cup common green cabbage (4)
¼ cup shredded red cabbage (5)
½ cup diced apples (28)
1 teaspoon canola oil (40)
Vinegar and spices of choice

Strawberry Smoothie
8 ounces sugar-free, nonfat yogurt (98)
1 cup strawberries (53)

1 borage oil capsule (taken with meal) (9)

DINNER—Pear-and-Cheese Salad (142), Roast Chicken, Corn-Bread Stuffing, Acorn Squash

Pear-and-Cheese Salad
2 pear halves (44)
2 ounces grated low-fat Cheddar cheese (98)

3 ounces roasted chicken breast (no skin) (147)
½ cup cornbread stuffing prepared from dry mix (179)
1 cup cooked acorn squash (83)
1 teaspoon trans-fat-free margarine (29)

1 borage oil capsule (taken with meal) (9)

SNACK—Celery with Peanut Butter

2 celery stalks (11)
2 tablespoons peanut butter (192)

DAY 12 Nutritional Values
Calories—1,993
Fiber (g)—32.63
GI = all<70
% Fat—37.32
% SFA—9.50
% MUFA—14.79
% PUFA—10.92
AA (mg)—70
EPA (mg)—10
Cholesterol (mg)—138

DAY 13

BREAKFAST—Shredded-Wheat Cereal with Milk and Blueberries, Cantaloupe Wedge with Cottage Cheese
1 cup bite-sized shredded-wheat cereal (167)
¾ cup 1% milk (77)
½ cup blueberries (41)
⅛ medium cantaloupe (23)
½ cup 1% cottage cheese (81)

1 borage oil capsule (taken with meal) (9)

LUNCH—Chef's Salad with Ranch Dressing (415), Crackers, Tropical Gelatin Salad (82)
Chef's Salad with Low-Fat Ranch Dressing
2 cups green leaf lettuce (17)
5 cherry tomatoes (15)
¼ cup sliced cucumbers (4)
¼ cup sliced mushrooms (4)
3 ounces extra-lean ham (111)
3 ounces low-fat cheese (148)
3 large black olives (15)
3 tablespoons low-fat ranch dressing (101)

5 whole-wheat crackers (89)

Tropical Gelatin Salad
¾ cup prepared sugar-free gelatin (14)
¼ cup mandarin oranges (23)
1 tablespoon chopped pecans (45)

1 borage oil capsule (taken with meal) (9)

DINNER—Mackerel Jambalaya* (393), Brown Rice, Broccoli
Mackerel Jambalaya
4 ounces cooked Atlantic mackerel (or another Category 1 fish) (297)
¼ cup chopped green peppers (5)
¼ cup chopped yellow peppers (6)
¼ cup chopped onions (17)
1 cup diced tomatoes (68)

1 cup cooked brown rice (216)

1 cup cooked broccoli (44)
4 teaspoons trans-fat-free margarine (116)

1 borage oil capsule (taken with meal) (9)

SNACK—Peach Crumble (240)
Peach Crumble
1 medium peach (38)
2 tablespoons oats (76)
1 tablespoon slivered almonds (39)
1 tablespoon trans-fat-free margarine (87)

DAY 13 Nutritional Values
Calories—2,011
Fiber (g)—32.38
GI = all<70
% Fat—36.98
% SFA—8.52
% MUFA—16.07
% PUFA—8.50
AA (mg)—60
EPA (mg)—580
Cholesterol (mg)—171

* You'll find recipes for items marked with an asterisk * in chapter 18.

DAY 14

BREAKFAST—Bagel with Lox and Cream Cheese, Cranapple Juice

1 medium oat-bran bagel (145)

3 ounces lox (smoked Chinook salmon) (100)

2 tablespoons low-fat cream cheese (69)

8 ounces low-calorie cranapple juice (46)

1 borage oil capsule (taken with meal) (9)

LUNCH—Pita Pizza (370), Grapes

Pita Pizza

1 (4-inch) whole-wheat pita (for pizza crust) (74)

¼ cup marinara sauce (36)

2 ounces diced Canadian-style bacon (89)

¼ cup chopped onion (17)

¼ cup sliced mushrooms (10)

2 ounces part-skim mozzarella cheese (144)

1½ cups grapes (166)

1 borage oil capsule (taken with meal) (9)

DINNER—Beef-and-Vegetable Teriyaki Stir-Fry (540), Pasta, Pudding with Raspberries

Beef-and-Vegetable Teriyaki Stir-Fry

4 ounces cooked beef flank steak (211)

2 tablespoons teriyaki sauce (marinade for steak) (30)

½ cup snow peas (42)

½ cup sliced sweet red pepper (10)

½ cup sliced carrots (25)

1 tablespoon peanut oil to stir-fry steak and vegetables (119)

2 tablespoons sesame seeds (103)

1 cup cooked whole-wheat pasta (174)

½ cup sugar-free, nonfat vanilla pudding (75)

½ cup raspberries (32)

1 borage oil capsule (taken with meal) (9)

SNACK—Mixed Nuts

⅓ cup dry-roasted mixed nuts (269)

DAY 14 Nutritional Values
Calories—2,013
Fiber (g)—27.96
GI = all<70
% Fat—37.12
% SFA—10.09
% MUFA—16.31
% PUFA—7.81
AA (mg)—40
EPA (mg)—160
Cholesterol (mg)—157

DAY 15

BREAKFAST—Cheese-and-Vegetable Omelet (142), Toast with Margarine and Jelly, Cherries
Cheese-and-Vegetable Omelet
½ cup cooked liquid egg substitute (105)
½ ounce low-fat cheese (25)
2 tablespoons chopped onion (8)
2 tablespoons chopped green peppers (4)

2 slices whole-wheat bread (138)
2 teaspoons trans-fat-free margarine (58)
2 tablespoons reduced- or no-sugar
   jelly (68)
1 cup cherries (52)

1 borage oil capsule (taken with meal) (9)

LUNCH—Chicken Salad Veronique (459), Rye Crackers, Baby Carrots, Tomato Juice
Chicken Salad Veronique
3 ounces cooked chicken breast
   (no skin) (147)
2 tablespoons no-cholesterol
   mayonnaise (206)
¼ cup halved grapes (28)
2 tablespoons slivered almonds (78)

2 rye wafers (73)
8 baby carrots (28)
6 ounces tomato juice (31)

1 borage oil capsule (taken with meal) (9)

DINNER—Grilled Salmon Dijon* (436), Mixed Wild and Brown Rice, Green Peas, Gelatin with Fruit (46)
Grilled Salmon Dijon
5 ounces grilled or broiled wild sockeye
   salmon (or another Category 1 fish) (306)
1 tablespoon canola oil (120)
1 tablespoon Dijon mustard (10)

½ cup cooked wild rice (83)
½ cup cooked brown rice (108)
½ tablespoon trans-fat-free margarine (43)
1 cup cooked green peas (125)

Sugar-Free Gelatin with Fruit
1 cup sugar-free gelatin (19)
¼ cup mixed fruit (27)

1 borage oil capsule (taken with meal) (9)

SNACK—Yogurt Crunch (88)
Yogurt Crunch
6 ounces sugar-free, nonfat yogurt (73)
2 tablespoons Fiber One cereal (15)

DAY 15 Nutritional Values
Calories—2,005
Fiber (g)—32.28
GI = all<70
% Fat—38.72
% SFA—8.14
% MUFA—14.01
% PUFA—5.60
AA (mg)—110
EPA (mg)—760
Cholesterol (mg)—203

---

* You'll find recipes for items marked with an asterisk * in chapter 18.

DAY 16

BREAKFAST—Whole-Wheat Pancakes with Bananas, Pecans, and Sugar-Free Syrup, Milk

3 (4-inch) whole-wheat pancakes made
   from mix with liquid egg substitute (275)
1 small banana (90)
2 tablespoons pecans (86)
2 tablespoons reduced calorie syrup (49)
1 cup 1% milk (102)

1 borage oil capsule (taken with meal) (9)

LUNCH—Lentil Soup (161), Antipasto Salad (436), Rye Crackers
Lentil Soup
1 cup fat-free chicken broth (12)
½ cup cooked lentils (115)
¼ cup chopped onions (17)
¼ cup diced carrots (13)
¼ cup diced celery (4)

Antipasto Salad
2 cups romaine lettuce (19)
2 ounces part-skim mozzarella cheese (171)
2 ounces beef salami (146)
5 cherry tomatoes (15)
5 large black olives (25)
½ tablespoon olive oil (60)
Vinegar and spices of choice

2 rye wafers (73)

1 borage oil capsule (taken with meal) (9)

DINNER—Grilled Flank Steak, Broiled Tomatoes Parmesan (83), Spinach, Roll with Margarine
6 ounces cooked beef flank steak (316)

Broiled Tomatoes Parmesan
2 plum tomatoes (22)
½ ounce grated Parmesan cheese (61)

1 cup cooked spinach (41)
½ tablespoon olive oil (60)
1 small whole-wheat roll (75)
1 teaspoon trans-fat-free margarine (29)

1 borage oil capsule (taken with meal) (9)

SNACK—Fresh Grapes
1 cup grapes (110)

DAY 16 Nutritional Values
Calories—2,013
Fiber (g)—29.36
GI = all<70
% Fat—38.90
% SFA—12.79
% MUFA—18.13
% PUFA—5.83
AA (mg)—80
EPA (mg)—0
Cholesterol (mg)—259

DAY 17

BREAKFAST—All-Bran Cereal with Strawberries and Milk, Muffin with Cheese
½ cup Kellogg's All-Bran cereal (78)
¾ cup strawberries (36)
1 cup 1% milk (102)
1 multigrain English muffin (155)
2 teaspoons trans-fat-free margarine (58)
1 ounce low-fat cheese (50)

1 borage oil capsule (taken with meal) (9)

LUNCH—Blue Cheese Burger (424), Three-Bean Salad (205)
Blue Cheese Burger
1 whole-wheat hamburger roll (114)
4 ounces cooked ground beef
    (95% lean) (194)
1 ounce blue cheese (100)
1 slice onion (16)

Three-Bean Salad
¼ cup canned green beans (7)
¼ cup canned chickpeas (71)
¼ cup canned wax beans (7)
1 tablespoon canola oil (120)
Vinegar and spices of choice

1 borage oil capsule (taken with meal) (9)

DINNER—Baked Ham, Cranberried Acorn Squash (68), Broccoli, Peach Yogurt Sundae (326)
4 ounces lean baked ham (185)

Cranberried Acorn Squash
½ cooked acorn squash (62)
2 tablespoons fresh chopped cranberries (6)

1 cup cooked broccoli (44)
1 teaspoon trans-fat-free margarine (29)

Peach Yogurt Sundae
1 cup sugar-free, nonfat frozen yogurt (199)
2 tablespoons chopped pecans (94)
½ cup peaches (33)

1 borage oil capsule (taken with meal) (9)

SNACK—Salmon Spread* (148) on Crackers
Salmon Spread
2 ounces canned pink salmon (79)
2 tablespoons reduced-fat cream cheese (69)
Herbs and spices of choice

4 whole-wheat crackers (71)

DAY 17 Nutritional Values
Calories—2,006
Fiber (g)—41.22
GI = all<70
% Fat—36.61
% SFA—11.31
% MUFA—16.00
% PUFA—7.55
AA (mg)—150
EPA (mg)—480
Cholesterol (mg)—250

* You'll find recipes for items marked with an asterisk* in chapter 18.

DAY 18

BREAKFAST—Bran Muffin with Margarine, Peach, Chocolate Milk

1 small low-fat oat-bran muffin (178)
1 teaspoon trans-fat-free margarine (29)
1 small peach (31)
6 ounces low-fat chocolate milk (118)

1 borage oil capsule (taken with meal) (9)

LUNCH—Ham-and-Cheese Sandwich (376), Pretzels

Ham-and-Cheese Sandwich
2 slices whole-wheat bread (138)
3 ounces extra-lean ham (111)
1 ounce low-fat cheese (50)
1 leaf lettuce (1)
2 slices tomatoes (7)
2 teaspoons no-cholesterol mayonnaise (69)

1 ounce whole-wheat pretzels (103)

1 borage oil capsule (taken with meal) (9)

DINNER—Shrimp, Scallops, and Clams Italiano with Pasta* (705), Tossed Salad with Dressing (41)

Shrimp, Scallops, and Clams Italiano
3 ounces cooked shrimp (84)
2 ounces cooked scallops (64)
2 ounces cooked clams (84)
½ cup diced tomatoes (34)
½ cup chopped green peppers (15)
2 tablespoons olive oil to sauté shellfish
    and vegetables (239)
1 cup cooked whole-wheat spaghetti (174)
1 ounce grated fresh Parmesan cheese (111)

Tossed Salad with Low-Fat Dressing
1 cup romaine lettuce (10)
3 cherry tomatoes (9)
2 tablespoons low-fat Italian dressing (22)

1 small whole-wheat roll (75)
1 teaspoon trans-fat-free margarine (29)

1 borage oil capsule (taken with meal) (9)

SNACK—Apple Crisp (200)

Apple Crisp
½ cup apple slices (29)
2 tablespoons oats (76)
2 tablespoons sliced almonds (66)
1 teaspoon trans-fat-free margarine (29)

DAY 18 Nutritional Values
Calories—2,012
Fiber (g)—29.76
GI = all<70
% Fat—37.08
% SFA—8.11
% MUFA—18.26
% PUFA—8.43
AA (mg)—130
EPA (mg)—320
Cholesterol (mg)—310

* You'll find recipes for items marked with an asterisk * in chapter 18.

DAY 19

BREAKFAST—Loaded Bagel (420), Grapefruit Juice
Loaded Bagel
1 medium oat-bran bagel (145)
2 teaspoons trans-fat-free margarine (58)
½ cup cooked liquid egg substitute (105)
2 slices lean cooked bacon (74)
¾ ounces low-fat cheese (38)

8 ounces pink grapefruit juice (96)

1 borage oil capsule (taken with meal) (9)

LUNCH—Salmon Pasta Salad* (431), Crackers, Marinated Cucumbers (56)
Salmon Pasta Salad
3 ounces canned pink salmon (118)
1 cup cooked whole-wheat macaroni (174)
¼ cup chopped green bell pepper (10)
2 tablespoons chopped celery (2)
2 tablespoons chopped onion (8)
1 tablespoon olive oil (119)
Lemon juice, herbs, and spices of choice

6 whole-wheat crackers (106)

Marinated Cucumbers
1 cup sliced cucumbers (16)
1 teaspoon canola oil (40)
Vinegar, dill, and spices of choice

1 borage oil capsule (taken with meal) (9)

DINNER—Roast Pork, Baked Sweet Potato, Brussels Sprouts, Vanilla Pudding with Raspberries
3 ounces cooked lean top loin pork
   roast (165)
1 medium baked sweet potato (103)
1 cup cooked brussels sprouts (56)
1½ tablespoons trans-fat-free margarine
   (130)
½ cup sugar-free, nonfat vanilla
   pudding (75)
¼ cup raspberries (16)

1 borage oil capsule (taken with meal) (9)

SNACK—½ Peanut-Butter-and-Jelly Sandwich (329)
½ Peanut-Butter-and-Jelly Sandwich
1 slice whole-wheat bread (69)
2 tablespoons peanut butter (192)
2 tablespoons reduced- or no-sugar
   jelly (68)

DAY 19 Nutritional Values
Calories—2,010
Fiber (g)—24.69
GI = all<70
% Fat—39.67
% SFA—8.20
% MUFA—19.30
% PUFA—9.40
AA (mg)—120
EPA (mg)—720
Cholesterol (mg)—139

* You'll find recipes for items marked with an asterisk* in chapter 18.

DAY 20

BREAKFAST—Oatmeal with Blueberries and Walnuts, Mozzarella Cheese Stick, Orange Juice

1 cup cooked oatmeal (145)

¼ cup blueberries (21)

2 tablespoons chopped English walnuts (98)

1 ounce part-skim mozzarella cheese stick (72)

6 ounces unsweetened orange juice (78)

1 borage oil capsule (taken with meal) (9)

DAY 20 Nutritional Values
Calories—2,016
Fiber (g)—35.77
GI = all<70
% Fat—37.60
% SFA—13.05
% MUFA—17.15
% PUFA—5.31
AA (mg)—90
EPA (mg)—0
Cholesterol (mg)—237

LUNCH—Greek Lamb Pita, Tomato-Bulgur Salad (173)

Greek Lamb Pita

1 (6-inch) whole-wheat pita (170)

3 ounces cooked lean leg of lamb (190)

½ cup diced cucumber (7)

2 ounces feta cheese (150)

2 tablespoons vinegar and oil salad dressing (144)

Tomato-Bulgur Salad

¼ cup cooked bulgur (38)

½ cup chopped tomatoes (16)

1 tablespoon olive oil (119)

Lemon juice, vinegar, and herbs of choice

1 borage oil capsule (taken with meal) (9)

DINNER—Baked Chicken, Brown Rice, Carrots, Cherries

3 ounces baked chicken breast (no skin) (147)

1 cup cooked brown rice (216)

1 cup cooked carrots (55)

1 tablespoon trans-fat-free margarine (87)

1 cup cherries (88)

1 borage oil capsule (taken with meal) (9)

SNACK—Peaches and Yogurt

8 ounces sugar-free, nonfat yogurt (98)

¾ cup sliced peaches (50)

DAY 21

BREAKFAST—English Muffin with Margarine and Jelly, Cottage Cheese and Strawberries, Apple Juice

1 multigrain English muffin (155)
2 teaspoons trans-fat-free margarine (58)
2 tablespoons reduced- or no-sugar jelly (68)
¾ cup 1% cottage cheese (122)
1 cup strawberries (49)
4 ounces unsweetened apple juice (58)

1 borage oil capsule (taken with meal) (9)

LUNCH—Fried Oyster Salad* with Ranch Dressing (424), Crackers, Melon

Fried Oyster Salad with Low-Fat Ranch Dressing
2 cups green leaf lettuce (17)
9 medium breaded and fried oysters (260)
¼ cup sliced red onions (12)
¼ cup low-fat ranch salad dressing (135)

6 whole-wheat crackers (106)

¾ cup cantaloupe (45)
¾ cup honeydew (48)

1 borage oil capsule (taken with meal) (9)

DINNER—Herb-Grilled Pork Chop, Cauliflower with Cheese Sauce (223), Green Beans, Pear and Cheddar Salad (109), Roll with Margarine

3 ounces cooked lean pork loin chop (145)

Cauliflower with Cheese Sauce
1½ cups cooked cauliflower (43)
¼ cup white sauce (92)
1 ounce low-fat cheese (50)
1 cup cooked green beans (38)

Pear-and-Cheddar Salad
1 cup pears (71)
¾ ounce grated low-fat Cheddar cheese (38)

1 small oat-bran roll (67)
1 teaspoon trans-fat-free margarine (29)

1 borage oil capsule (taken with meal) (9)

SNACK—Crackers with Artificial Crab Salad* (163)

6 whole-wheat crackers (106)

Artificial Crab Salad
2 ounces imitation crabmeat (surimi) (58)
1 tablespoon no-cholesterol mayonnaise (103)
2 tablespoons minced celery (2)

DAY 21 Nutritional Values
Calories—2,002
Fiber (g)—29.27
GI = all<70
% Fat—35.86
% SFA—8.04
% MUFA—12.73
% PUFA—11.05
AA (mg)—150
EPA (mg)—400
Cholesterol (mg)—219

---

* You'll find recipes for items marked with an asterisk* in chapter 18.

DAY 22

BREAKFAST—Scrambled Egg Substitute, English Muffin with Margarine and Jelly, Cranapple Juice

½ cup cooked liquid egg substitute (105)
1 multigrain English muffin (155)
2 teaspoons trans-fat-free margarine (58)
2 tablespoons reduced- or no-sugar
  jelly (68)
8 ounces low-calorie cranapple juice (46)

1 borage oil capsule (taken with meal) (9)

LUNCH—Chili Con Carne (269), Crackers, Fresh Apple

Chili Con Carne
2 ounces cooked ground beef
  (95% lean) (97)
½ cup cooked kidney beans (104)
1 cup canned, diced tomatoes (68)

2 ounces low-fat Cheddar cheese (98)
6 whole-wheat crackers (106)
1 medium apple (72)

1 borage oil capsule (taken with meal) (9)

DINNER—Scallop-and-Asparagus Sauté with Pasta* (588), Chocolate Pudding with Raspberries

Scallop-and-Asparagus Sauté
8 ounces cooked scallops (254)
1 cup cooked asparagus (40)
1 tablespoon canola oil to sauté scallops and
  asparagus (120)
1 cup cooked whole-wheat pasta (174)

½ cup sugar-free, nonfat chocolate
  pudding (74)
¼ cup raspberries (16)

1 borage oil capsule (taken with meal) (9)

SNACK—Peanuts

2 ounces dry-roasted peanuts (332)

DAY 22 Nutritional Values
Calories—2,014
Fiber (g)—30.47
GI = all<70
% Fat—32.77
% SFA—5.89
% MUFA—14.24
% PUFA—9.73
AA (mg)—120
EPA (mg)—380
Cholesterol (mg)—176

* You'll find recipes for items marked with an asterisk * in chapter 18.

DAY 23

BREAKFAST—Toast with Almond Butter and Sliced Apple, Milk
2 slices whole-wheat bread (138)
1 tablespoon almond butter (101)
1 medium apple, sliced (72)
1 cup 1% milk (102)

1 borage oil capsule (taken with meal) (9)

LUNCH—Curried Chicken Salad (465), Fruit Salad (93)
Curried Chicken Salad
3 ounces cooked chicken breast
   (no skin) (147)
½ cup cooked brown rice (108)
2 tablespoons no-cholesterol
   mayonnaise (206)
¼ cup diced celery (4)
Curry powder, lemon juice, and spices
   of choice

Fruit Salad
¼ cup sliced peaches (17)
¼ cup grapes (28)
¼ cup blueberries (21)
¼ cup kiwi (27)

1 borage oil capsule (taken with meal) (9)

DINNER—Baked Salmon* (306), Corn Bread Stuffing, Snow Peas, Apricot Crisp (139)
5 ounces baked sockeye salmon (or another
   Category 1 fish) (306)
1 cup corn bread stuffing, prepared from
   mix (358)
1 cup cooked snow peas (83)
Sliced green onions

Apricot Crisp
2 apricots (34)
2 tablespoons oats (76)
1 teaspoons trans-fat-free margarine (29)

1 borage oil capsule (taken with meal) (9)

SNACK—Cheese-and-Pepper Pita Toasts (129)
Cheese-and-Pepper Pita Toasts
1 (4-inch) whole-wheat pita (74)
1 ounce low-fat Cheddar cheese (49)
¼ cup chopped sweet red peppers (6)

DAY 23 Nutritional Values
Calories—2,013
Fiber (g)—30.13
GI = all<70
% Fat—38.48
% SFA—7.44
% MUFA—15.29
% PUFA—13.15
AA (mg)—110
EPA (mg)—760
Cholesterol (mg)—214

---

* You'll find recipes for items marked with an asterisk * in chapter 18.

DAY 24

BREAKFAST—Yogurt with Blueberries, Oatmeal Muffin with Margarine, Milk

8 ounces sugar-free, nonfat yogurt (98)
½ cup blueberries (41)
1 medium low-fat bran muffin (169)
1 teaspoon trans-fat-free margarine (29)
1 cup 1% milk (102)

1 borage oil capsule (taken with meal) (9)

LUNCH—Steak-and-Blue-Cheese Salad (426), Roll with Margarine, Fresh Kiwi

Steak-and-Blue-Cheese Salad
2 cups green leaf lettuce (17)
3 ounces cooked beef flank steak (158)
1 ounce blue cheese (100)
¼ cup sliced carrots (11)
¼ cup sliced onions (12)
3 tablespoons Italian salad dressing (128)

1 small whole-wheat roll (74)
1 teaspoon trans-fat-free margarine (29)
1 kiwi fruit (56)

1 borage oil capsule (taken with meal) (9)

DINNER—Roasted Herb Chicken, Wild Rice, Summer Squash, Frozen Yogurt with Bananas

4 ounces cooked chicken breast
   (no skin) (196)
1 cup cooked wild rice (166)
1 cup cooked summer squash (36)
1 tablespoon trans-fat-free margarine (87)
1 cup sugar-free, nonfat yogurt (199)
½ cup sliced banana (67)

1 borage oil capsule (taken with meal) (9)

SNACK—Celery Stuffed with Peanut Butter

2 stalks celery (11)
2 tablespoons peanut butter (192)

DAY 24 Nutritional Values
Calories—2,005
Fiber (g)—25.47
GI = all<70
% Fat—36.15
% SFA—10.15
% MUFA—13.36
% PUFA—9.59
AA (mg)—130
EPA (mg)—10
Cholesterol (mg)—206

DAY 25

BREAKFAST—Oatmeal with Milk and Strawberries, Orange Juice
1 cup cooked oatmeal (145)
¾ cup strawberries (40)
1 cup 1% milk (102)
8 ounces unsweetened orange juice (105)

1 borage oil capsule (taken with meal) (9)

LUNCH—Roast Beef, Swiss, and Cucumber Sandwich (443), Corn-and-Black-Bean Salad (260), Fresh Plum
Roast Beef, Swiss, and Cucumber Sandwich
2 slices oat bran (142)
3 ounces cooked lean eye of round beef (143)
1 ounce low-fat Swiss cheese (50)
6 cucumber slices (5)
1 tablespoon no-cholesterol mayonnaise (103)

Corn-and-Black-Bean Salad
⅓ cup cooked yellow corn (58)
⅓ cup canned black beans (72)
¼ cup chopped sweet red pepper (10)
1 tablespoon canola oil (120)
Lemon juice, vinegar, cilantro, and spices of choice

1 plum (30)

1 borage oil capsule (taken with meal) (9)

DINNER—Lemon-Herb Mackerel* (339), Carrots, Green Beans, Blueberries with Vanilla Yogurt
5 ounces broiled or grilled mackerel (or another Category 1 fish) (339)
1 cup cooked carrots (55)
1 cup cooked green beans (38)
1 tablespoon trans-fat-free margarine (87)
8 ounces sugar-free, nonfat vanilla yogurt (98)
¾ cup blueberries (62)

1 borage oil capsule (taken with meal) (9)

SNACK—Crackers with Low-Fat Cheese
2 rye wafers (73)
2 ounces low-fat cheese (98)

DAY 25 Nutritional Values
Calories—2,002
Fiber (g)—34.99
GI = all<70
% Fat—36.64
% SFA—7.78
% MUFA—17.02
% PUFA—9.04
AA (mg)—130
EPA (mg)—960
Cholesterol (mg)—181

* You'll find recipes for items marked with an asterisk * in chapter 18.

DAY 26

BREAKFAST—Waffles with Margarine, Sugar-Free Syrup, and Apples
2 (7-inch) whole-grain waffles (436)
2 teaspoons trans-fat-free margarine (58)
2 tablespoons reduced calorie pancake syrup (49)
1 cup unsweetened apples (97)

1 borage oil capsule (taken with meal) (9)

LUNCH—Crab Omelet (245), Toast with Margarine, Fresh Orange
Crab Omelet
½ cup cooked liquid egg substitute (105)
3 ounces cooked Alaskan-king-crab meat (82)
¼ cup diced green peppers (8)
¼ cup diced sweet red peppers (10)
1 teaspoon canola oil (40)

1 slice oatmeal bread (73)
1 teaspoon trans-fat-free margarine (29)
1 orange (62)

1 borage oil capsule (taken with meal) (9)

DINNER—Spaghetti with Meat Sauce (532), Tossed Salad with Italian Dressing (47), Roll with Margarine, Strawberry-Almond-Ricotta Parfait (227)
Spaghetti with Meat Sauce
1 cup cooked whole-wheat spaghetti (174)
4 ounces cooked ground beef (95% lean) (194)
1 cup marinara sauce (142)
1 tablespoon grated Parmesan cheese (22)

Tossed Salad with Italian Dressing
1 cup romaine lettuce (10)
5 cherry tomatoes (15)
2 tablespoons low-fat Italian salad dressing (22)

1 small whole-wheat roll (75)
1 teaspoon trans-fat-free margarine (29)

Strawberry-Almond-Ricotta Parfait
½ cup low-fat ricotta cheese (170)
½ cup strawberries (24)
2 tablespoons sliced almonds (33)

1 borage oil capsule (taken with meal) (9)

SNACK—Baby Carrots
5 baby carrots (18)

DAY 26 Nutritional Values
Calories—2,004
Fiber (g)—27.10
GI = all<70
% Fat—35.60
% SFA—9.42
% MUFA—13.06
% PUFA—10.64
AA (mg)—50
EPA (mg)—0
Cholesterol (mg)—280

DAY 27

BREAKFAST—Muesli Cereal with Milk and Peaches, Mozzarella Cheese Stick, Orange Juice

¾ cup muesli cereal (217)

1 cup 1% milk (102)

1 small peach (31)

1 ounce part-skim mozzarella cheese stick (86)

4 ounces unsweetened orange juice (52)

1 borage oil capsule (taken with meal) (9)

LUNCH—Beef Reuben Sandwich (440), Macaroni Salad (307)

Beef Reuben Sandwich

2 slices pumpernickel bread (130)

4 ounces cooked lean eye of round beef (191)

¼ cup sauerkraut (8)

1 ounce low-fat Swiss cheese (50)

2 tablespoons reduced-fat thousand island dressing (61)

Macaroni Salad

½ cup cooked macaroni (99)

2 tablespoons no-cholesterol mayonnaise (206)

2 tablespoons diced celery (2)

1 borage oil capsule (taken with meal) (9)

DINNER—Shrimp Creole* (322), Brown Rice, Stewed Okra and Tomatoes

Shrimp Creole

5 ounces cooked shrimp (140)

¼ cup chopped celery (4)

¼ cup chopped green pepper (8)

¼ cup chopped onions (17)

½ cup peeled and chopped tomatoes (34)

1 tablespoon olive oil to sauté vegetables (119)

1 cup cooked brown rice (216)

⅓ cup cooked okra (9)

⅓ cup cooked tomatoes (14)

1 borage oil capsule (taken with meal) (9)

SNACK—Chocolate, Hazelnut, and Banana Sandwich (186)

Chocolate, Hazelnut, and Banana Sandwich

1 slice whole-wheat bread (69)

1 tablespoon chocolate-flavored hazelnut spread (100)

2 tablespoons sliced banana (17)

DAY 27 Nutritional Values

Calories—2,009

Fiber (g)—23.73

GI = all<70

% Fat—32.87

% SFA—7.53

% MUFA—13.34

% PUFA—9.73

AA (mg)—120

EPA (mg)—240

Cholesterol (mg)—392

---

* You'll find recipes for items marked with an asterisk * in chapter 18.

DAY 28

BREAKFAST—English Muffin with Cheese, Citrus Sections

1 multigrain English muffin (155)
2 teaspoons trans-fat-free margarine (58)
1½ ounces low-fat cheese (76)
½ cup grapefruit sections (37)
½ cup orange sections (42)

1 borage oil capsule (taken with meal) (9)

LUNCH—Grilled Salmon Salad* (476), Bread, Grapes

Grilled Salmon Salad

2 cups green leaf lettuce (17)
5 ounces grilled or broiled sockeye salmon
    (or another Category 1 fish) (306)
¼ cup sliced cucumbers (4)
¼ cup sliced carrots (13)
¼ cup sliced onions (17)
1 tablespoon olive oil (119)
Vinegar, herbs, and spices of choice

1 slice whole-wheat bread (69)
2 cups grapes (221)

1 borage oil capsule (taken with meal) (9)

DINNER—Grilled Pork Tenderloin, Sweet Potato, Broccoli with Cheese Sauce (234), Roll with Margarine

5 ounces grilled pork tenderloin (232)
1 medium baked sweet potato (103)
1 teaspoon trans-fat-free margarine (29)

Broccoli with Cheese Sauce

1 cup cooked broccoli (44)
¼ cup white sauce (92)
2 ounces low-fat Cheddar cheese (98)

1 small whole-wheat roll (75)
1 teaspoon trans-fat-free margarine (29)

1 borage oil capsule (taken with meal) (9)

SNACK—Berry Smoothie (147)

Berry Smoothie

8 ounces sugar-free, nonfat yogurt (98)
¼ cup strawberries (12)
¼ cup raspberries (16)
¼ cup blueberries (21)

DAY 28 Nutritional Values
Calories—2,010
Fiber (g)—28.06
GI = all<70
% Fat—31.26
% SFA—7.62
% MUFA—15.33
% PUFA—5.76
AA (mg)—90
EPA (mg)—750
Cholesterol (mg)—271

* You'll find recipes for items marked with an asterisk * in chapter 18.

Chapter Eighteen

Inflammation Nation Seafood Recipes

The recipes that follow correspond to the menu items in the meal plans that are marked with asterisks. Each recipe yields two servings.

What's important to me is the type of fish—Category 1, 2, or 3—that you use, not the seasonings or cooking methods, so please feel free to use these as a jumping-off point for your own culinary creations.

Enjoy!

Crab Cakes
Prevention Diet, Day 21
Solution Diet, Day 5

12 ounces cooked or canned crabmeat
¼ cup liquid egg substitute
½ cup dry bread crumbs (divided)
1 tablespoon prepared mustard
1 teaspoon Worcestershire sauce
Salt and pepper to taste
Garlic powder to taste
¼ cup canola oil

Mix crabmeat, egg substitute, ¼ cup bread crumbs, and seasonings. Form into 4 cakes. Roll each cake in remaining bread crumbs. Heat oil in skillet. Fry cakes approximately 5 minutes on each side or just until well browned.

Artificial Crab (Surimi) Salad

Prevention Diet, Day 8
Solution Diet, Day 21

    4 to 6 ounces artificial crabmeat (surimi)
    2 tablespoons no-cholesterol mayonnaise
    1 tablespoon lemon juice
    2 to 4 tablespoons minced celery

Combine all ingredients. Cover and chill 2 hours. Serve with crackers.

Crabmeat Lasagna Rolls

Prevention Diet, Day 13

    4 whole-wheat lasagna noodles, uncooked
    8 ounces canned blue-crab meat
    ½ cup 1% cottage cheese
    1 tablespoon dried parsley flakes
    ¼ teaspoon onion powder
    ¼ teaspoon black pepper
    1 cup marinara sauce
    ¼ cup grated Parmesan cheese

Cook noodles as directed on package. Rinse under cold water; drain well.

Combine crabmeat, cottage cheese, and seasonings. Lay noodles out flat on work surface and spread one-fourth of filling over each noodle. Roll as tightly as possible. Place seam-side down in a baking dish that has been sprayed with nonstick cooking spray. Pour pasta sauce over roll-ups. Cover dish and bake at 375°F for 30 minutes. Sprinkle with Parmesan cheese and return to oven, uncovered, for 5 minutes to melt cheese.

Lemon-Herb Mackerel or Salmon

Prevention Diet, Day 10
Solution Diet, Days 1, 7, 25

    12 ounces fresh or frozen wild mackerel or salmon filets
    2 tablespoons lemon juice
    2 tablespoons chopped fresh parsley
    ¼ teaspoon dill weed
    ¼ teaspoon salt
    ⅛ teaspoon coarsely ground black pepper

Line broiler pan with aluminum foil and spray broiler rack with nonstick coating spray. Place fish filets on rack. Combine remaining ingredients; baste fish with mixture. Broil 4 inches from heat, allowing 10 minutes per inch of thickness measured at thickest point or until fish flakes easily with fork. Do not turn. Baste several times during cooking time. Serve immediately.

Mackerel-and-Crab Jambalaya

Prevention Diet, Day 15
Solution Diet, Day 13

    ½ cup chopped green and/or yellow onion
    ½ cup chopped green bell pepper
    ½ cup chopped yellow bell pepper
    2 stalks celery with leaves, chopped
    ½ teaspoon minced garlic
    8 ounces fresh, frozen, or canned Atlantic mackerel
    4 ounces fresh, frozen, or canned crabmeat
    2 cups canned diced tomatoes
    2 cups defatted chicken broth
    ½ teaspoon salt
    ¼ teaspoon cayenne pepper
    ⅓ cup uncooked brown rice

In a large skillet coated with nonstick cooking spray, sauté onion, peppers, celery, and garlic until tender but not brown. Chop mackerel and crabmeat, add to skillet, and cook 5 minutes. Add tomatoes, broth, salt, cayenne, and rice. Stir, cover, and cook 30 to 40 minutes over low heat or until rice is done. If mixture becomes too dry, tomato juice may be added.

Fried Oyster Salad
Solution Diet, Day 21

> ¼ cup yellow cornmeal or finely grated bread crumbs
> Black pepper, cayenne pepper, and salt to taste
> 10 ounces (about 18) shucked oysters, drained
> ¼ cup canola oil
> 4 cups torn green leaf lettuce or other salad greens
> ½ cup sliced red onions
> ½ cup ranch salad dressing (divided)

Place cornmeal, peppers, and salt in a plastic bag. Place oysters, 6 at a time, in bag and shake to coat completely. Tap oysters to remove excess coating. In a heavy skillet, heat oil to 375°F. Fry oysters, 6 at a time, turning occasionally until golden brown. Place on paper towels to drain. Divide greens into two salad bowls. Add onions (and other salad vegetables of choice) and top each salad with 9 fried oysters. Serve with ¼ cup reduced fat ranch salad dressing per serving.

Scalloped Oysters
Prevention Diet, Day 23

> ½ cup bread crumbs (divided)
> ¼ cup trans-fat-free margarine, melted
> 10 ounces eastern oysters (about 30 medium), drained (reserving ¼ cup liquid)
> Salt and pepper to taste

Preheat oven to 450°F. Mix ¼ cup bread crumbs with melted margarine to form crumbles. Place in a shallow baking dish that has been sprayed with nonstick cooking spray. Place half of the oysters on top of the bread crumbles. Season with salt and pepper. Sprinkle with half of the reserved oyster liquid. Repeat with one more layer. Top with remaining bread crumbs. Bake for 30 minutes.

Salmon Cakes
Prevention Diet, Day 6

> 6 ounces canned pink salmon
> ¼ cup liquid egg substitute
> ½ tablespoon Dijon mustard
> ¼ cup dry bread crumbs
> 3 tablespoons finely chopped onion
> ¼ teaspoon garlic salt
> ¼ cup canola oil

Drain salmon. Remove any bones and flake salmon into bowl. Add egg substitute, mustard, and bread crumbs; mix well. Stir in onion and garlic salt. Heat oil in skillet. Drop mixture into skillet by ¼-cup amounts; flatten. Cook on one side, then flip and cook on other side until brown on both sides.

Salmon in Sun-Dried-Tomato Cream Sauce
Prevention Diet, Day 26

> ½ cup sun-dried tomatoes
> 2 cloves fresh garlic, minced
> 2 tablespoons trans-fat-free margarine
> 2 tablespoons flour
> ¼ teaspoon salt
> ¼ teaspoon black pepper
> 1 cup fat-free half-and-half
> 8 ounces cooked wild sockeye or canned pink salmon
> ½ cup chopped fresh basil
> 2 cups cooked whole-wheat pasta
> 2 ounces (¾ cup) grated fresh Parmesan cheese

Place sun-dried tomatoes in a bowl. Pour boiling water over tomatoes and allow to soak while making white sauce. In a skillet coated with non-stick cooking spray, sauté garlic until browned. Add margarine and melt it, being careful not to scorch. Blend in flour, salt, and pepper. Cook over low heat, stirring constantly, until smooth and bubbly; remove from heat. Stir in half-and-half. Heat to boiling, stirring constantly. Reduce heat. Drain tomatoes and chop; stir into sauce. Flake salmon; add it and basil to sauce. Heat gently for 2 minutes. Serve over 2 cups whole-wheat pasta, cooked per package directions. Top with Parmesan cheese.

Grilled Salmon Teriyaki
Prevention Diet, Day 1

2 (8-ounce) salmon filets
2 tablespoons reduced sodium teriyaki sauce
½ teaspoon coarsely ground black pepper

Place salmon in a bowl or shallow dish. Pour teriyaki sauce over filets; cover and let stand for 10 minutes at room temperature. Spray grill with nonstick cooking spray and heat to 450°F. Remove salmon from marinade. Rub pepper into skinless side of each filet. Place salmon on grill, skin-side up, and cook over medium-high (400°F) heat for 3 to 4 minutes. Turn and cook 2 minutes more. Serve immediately.

Broiled Salmon
Solution Diet, Day 3

1 pound wild sockeye salmon
Freshly ground black pepper
1 teaspoon minced fresh ginger
1 teaspoon minced garlic
Salt to taste
¼ teaspoon white pepper
¼ cup lemon juice
¼ cup white vinegar

Season salmon with black pepper to taste. Refrigerate until ready to use. Combine ginger, garlic, salt, white pepper, lemon juice, and vinegar in a saucepan. Boil 2 to 3 minutes. Remove from heat; let cool. Preheat oven to 450°F. Brush salmon with prepared marinade. Broil quickly until it feels springy to the touch, about 5 minutes per side.

Salmon Pasta Salad
Solution Diet, Day 19

6 ounces canned pink salmon

2 cups whole-wheat macaroni (about 1 cup uncooked),
  cooked per package directions

½ cup chopped green bell pepper

¼ cup chopped celery

¼ cup chopped red onion

¼ cup lemon juice

2 tablespoons olive oil

2 tablespoons chopped fresh basil (or 2 teaspoons dried)

⅛ teaspoon salt

¼ teaspoon black pepper

Garlic powder to taste

Combine all ingredients in a bowl. Cover and refrigerate at least 8 hours.

Grilled Salmon Dijon
Solution Diet, Day 15

2 tablespoons Dijon mustard

1 tablespoon lemon juice

2 tablespoons canola oil

2 (6-ounce) wild sockeye salmon filets

Combine mustard, lemon juice, and oil. Spray heavy-duty aluminum pan with nonstick cooking spray. Place salmon skin-side down on foil. Brush sauce over salmon. Form a tent over salmon with another piece of foil;

seal edges. Grill over medium heat for 8 to 15 minutes, depending on thickness, or until salmon flakes easily with a fork. Total cooking time should be 10 minutes per inch of thickness at the thickest point.

Greek Salmon Salad
Solution Diet, Day 10

Dressing
2 tablespoons olive oil
2 tablespoons lemon juice
¼ teaspoon garlic salt
Pinch of coarsely ground black pepper
Pinch of crushed oregano leaves

4 cups torn romaine lettuce or other salad greens
½ cup sliced cucumbers
8 large black olives, sliced (¼ cup)
¼ cup chopped green onions
1 cup chopped fresh Roma tomatoes
8 ounces grilled or baked wild sockeye or canned pink salmon
2 ounces feta cheese

In a small bowl, whisk together dressing ingredients until well blended. Refrigerate until ready to serve. Place lettuce in bowl or on serving platter. Top with cucumbers, olives, green onions, and tomatoes. Flake salmon (removing bones if using canned salmon) over the top of the vegetables. Crumble feta cheese over top. Drizzle dressing over salad and serve immediately.

Salmon Spread
Solution Diet, Day 17

4 ounces canned pink salmon, drained
4 tablespoons reduced fat cream cheese

1 teaspoon Dijon mustard

1 tablespoon chopped fresh parsley

⅛ teaspoon black pepper

⅛ teaspoon cayenne pepper

Combine all ingredients. Cover and chill at least 2 hours. Serve on crackers.

Baked Salmon
Solution Diet, Day 23

2 (6-ounce) sockeye salmon steaks

¼ cup green onions with tops, sliced

¼ cup dry white wine

1 teaspoon fresh dill weed

¼ teaspoon black pepper

Place salmon in a baking dish. Add remaining ingredients and cover. Place in refrigerator for 30 minutes, turning once during that time. Remove from refrigerator and allow to stand at room temperature for 20 minutes. Preheat oven to 350°F. Bake for 30 to 35 minutes, basting with marinade during cooking. Fish is done when it flakes easily with a fork.

Seafood Pasta Salad
Prevention Diet, Day 17

4 ounces canned blue-crab meat

4 ounces cooked peeled and deveined shrimp, tails removed

2 cups cooked small shell pasta

1 cup asparagus cuts, blanched

6 tablespoons no-cholesterol mayonnaise

2 tablespoons chopped fresh dill

1 teaspoon lemon zest

Salt and black pepper to taste

Juice of 1 lemon

Flake crabmeat and chop shrimp. In a bowl, combine all ingredients except lemon juice. Toss together well. Cover and refrigerate 2 hours. Before serving add lemon juice and adjust seasonings. Serve immediately.

Shrimp Chowder
Prevention Diet, Day 8

¼ cup trans-fat-free margarine

¼ cup chopped onion

¼ cup flour

2 cups 1% milk

½ to ¾ cup defatted chicken broth

1 cup fresh or frozen corn

8 ounces cooked peeled and deveined shrimp, tails removed

1 teaspoon dried basil

Salt and pepper to taste

Melt margarine in saucepan. Sauté onion until golden. Add flour and stir continuously until smooth and bubbly. Add milk and cook over medium heat, stirring continuously, until thickened. Add broth, corn, shrimp, and seasonings. Cook over low heat just until heated through.

Curried Shrimp Salad
Prevention Diet, Day 24

1⅓ cups water

½ teaspoon salt

⅔ cup uncooked long-grain brown rice

6 tablespoons no-cholesterol mayonnaise dressing

1 tablespoon lemon juice

2 teaspoons curry powder

2 tablespoons grated onion

10 ounces cooked peeled and deveined shrimp, tails removed
    (approximately 2¼ cups chopped)

⅔ cup frozen peas, thawed

Bring water to a boil. Stir in salt and rice; reduce heat. Simmer, covered, until done (30 to 40 minutes). Fluff lightly with a fork, and then cool to room temperature. Combine remaining ingredients; mix in rice and chill.

Grilled Shrimp
Prevention Diet, Day 28

- 4 teaspoons canola oil
- 2 cloves garlic, minced
- 2 tablespoons chopped fresh parsley
- 12 ounces fresh or frozen shrimp

Whisk oil, garlic, and parsley vigorously to blend well. Peel and devein shrimp. Divide shrimp onto two pieces of heavy-duty aluminum foil. Divide sauce evenly over shrimp. Fold and secure foil tightly at edges. Grill foil packets over medium heat for 10 to 12 minutes.

Shrimp-and-Scallops Scampi
Prevention Diet, Day 18

- 2 tablespoons olive oil
- 2 cloves garlic, minced
- ½ teaspoon dried oregano
- ½ teaspoon dried basil
- ¼ teaspoon crushed red pepper flakes
- ½ cup defatted chicken broth
- 6 ounces peeled and deveined shrimp
- 6 ounces fresh or frozen scallops
- ½ fresh lemon

In a large skillet heat oil over medium-high heat; add garlic. Cook until browned, about 3 minutes. Add oregano, basil, red pepper flakes, and broth to skillet; stir. Bring sauce to a simmer; cook 3 minutes. Add shrimp and scallops to skillet and cook just until shrimp turn firm and pink (about 3 to 5 minutes). Squeeze lemon juice over top and serve immediately.

Shrimp-and-Vegetable Stir-Fry I
Prevention Diet, Day 4

¼ cup olive oil (divided)

1 tablespoon minced fresh garlic

12 ounces fresh or frozen shrimp, peeled and deveined

1 cup diced celery

1 cup diced green bell pepper

1 cup diced tomatoes

2 cups cooked whole-wheat spaghetti

In a large skillet heat 2 tablespoons of the oil over medium-high heat. Add garlic and shrimp. Cook 5 minutes, or until the shrimp turn pink, stirring constantly. Transfer shrimp to a plate. In same skillet, heat remaining oil. Add celery and pepper and cook 2 minutes, stirring constantly, until crisp-tender. Stir in tomatoes and shrimp; cook until heated through. Serve over cooked spaghetti.

Shrimp-and-Vegetable Stir-Fry II
Solution Diet, Day 11

Juice and zest of 1 lemon

1 tablespoon Dijon mustard

1 clove garlic, crushed

1 cup red onion, thinly sliced

2 tablespoons olive oil (divided)

Salt and pepper to taste

8 ounces fresh or frozen shrimp, peeled and deveined

1 cup sliced red bell pepper

1 cup snow pea pods

2 cups cherry tomatoes, halved

2 cups cooked whole-wheat spaghetti

In a bowl combine lemon juice, zest, mustard, garlic, and onion. Add 1 tablespoon olive oil and whisk until thoroughly blended. Add salt and pepper to taste. Add shrimp to dressing and toss. Cover and refrigerate

6 to 8 hours. Before serving time, heat remaining oil in a skillet that has been coated with nonstick cooking spray. Sauté red pepper and snow pea pods until crisp-tender. Remove shrimp from marinade, reserving marinade, and add to skillet. Cook, stirring frequently, for 3 to 5 minutes or until shrimp are pink. Add tomatoes and reserved marinade; heat through. Serve over cooked spaghetti.

Shrimp, Scallops, and Clams Italiano
Solution Diet, Day 18

> 6 ounces peeled and deveined shrimp
>
> 4 ounces fresh or frozen scallops
>
> 4 ounces fresh, frozen, or canned clams
>
> ¼ cup olive oil
>
> 4 cloves garlic, minced
>
> 1 cup chopped green bell pepper
>
> 1 cup canned or fresh diced tomatoes
>
> Salt and pepper to taste
>
> 2 tablespoons chopped fresh parsley
>
> 2 cups whole-wheat spaghetti, cooked per package instructions
>
> 2 ounces (¾ cup) grated fresh Parmesan cheese

Poach shrimp and scallops (and clams if using fresh or frozen uncooked) about 3 to 5 minutes in a medium saucepan of boiling water, reserving ½ cup of the liquid after cooking. Drain shellfish and keep warm. Heat the oil in a large skillet over medium heat. Add garlic and peppers and sauté until crisp-tender. Add tomatoes, reserved shellfish liquid, salt, pepper, and parsley; boil gently for 5 minutes. Add the shellfish to the tomato sauce, reduce heat to low, and simmer gently for 5 minutes. Place cooked pasta in hot serving dish. Add sauce and mix well. Top with Parmesan cheese.

Scallop-and-Asparagus Sauté

Solution Diet, Day 22

1 cup uncooked whole-wheat pasta

2 cups asparagus stalks (about 16 medium), cut in 3–4" lengths

2 tablespoons canola oil

1 pound scallops

1 cup fish stock

1 tablespoon cornstarch

Juice of 2 lemons

Salt and pepper to taste

Cook pasta according to package directions. Drain and keep warm. Meanwhile steam asparagus until crisp-tender; drain and set aside. Heat oil in skillet. Sauté scallops for 2 to 3 minutes. (Note: scallops are a delicate seafood and require very little cooking time. Be careful not to overcook.) In a small saucepan, stir ¼ cup of the fish stock with cornstarch, removing all lumps. Add remaining stock and bring to a boil over medium-high heat, stirring continuously until slightly thickened. Reduce heat. Add lemon juice, salt, and pepper, and simmer while preparing serving plates. Place cooked pasta on two plates. Divide asparagus and scallops evenly over the pasta. Pour sauce over each. Serve immediately.

Shrimp Creole

Solution Diet, Day 27

2 tablespoons olive oil

½ cup celery, chopped

½ cup green pepper, chopped

½ cup onion, chopped

2 cloves garlic, chopped

1 cup tomatoes, peeled and chopped

¾ cup water

2 teaspoons Worcestershire sauce

¼ teaspoon salt

¼ teaspoon black pepper

⅛ teaspoon cayenne pepper

¼ teaspoon hot pepper sauce

1 bay leaf

½ teaspoon crushed thyme

2 tablespoons chopped parsley

1 packet sugar substitute

12 ounces peeled and deveined shrimp

Heat oil in skillet. Sauté celery, peppers, onion, and garlic in oil until crisp-tender. Add tomatoes, water, and seasonings. Cook slowly, stirring occasionally, for 20 to 30 minutes. (Sauce may be prepared a day in advance.) Coat a sauté pan with nonstick cooking spray. Add shrimp and sauté until pink. Before serving, add shrimp to sauce and heat through. Serve over brown rice.

Tuna Salad
Solution Diet, Day 11

6 ounces white tuna, packed in water

4 teaspoons no-cholesterol mayonnaise

¼ cup finely chopped celery

Salt and pepper top taste

Combine all ingredients. Cover and refrigerate 2 hours.

Grilled Tuna or Salmon for Salad
Solution Diet, Days 9 and 28

6 ounces fresh or frozen wild bluefin tuna or sockeye salmon steaks

2 tablespoons lemon juice

2 garlic cloves, minced

Thaw fish if frozen. Place in a shallow bowl. Combine lemon juice and garlic; pour over fish. Refrigerate 1 hour, turning once. Remove fish from marinade and grill on medium-hot grill 5 to 6 minutes per side, depending on thickness. Steaks are done when pink in center. Prepare salad with greens and vegetables of choice. Place warm fish steaks atop and serve with dressing.

Tuna Melt Sandwich
Prevention Diet, Day 20

- 6 ounces canned white tuna, packed in water
- 2 tablespoons no-cholesterol mayonnaise
- ¼ cup chopped green onion
- ¼ teaspoon ground cumin
- ⅛ teaspoon black pepper
- 2 mixed-grain English muffins, split
- 4 ounces reduced-fat Swiss cheese, in slices

Mix drained and flaked tuna with mayonnaise, onion, cumin, and pepper. Top each muffin half with one-quarter of the tuna mixture. Place on cookie sheet. Broil for 1 minute. Top each muffin half with 1 ounce sliced Swiss cheese. Broil 1 to 2 minutes more or until cheese begins to melt and brown.

Tuna Pasta Salad
Prevention Diet, Day 3

- 6 ounces white tuna, canned in water
- 2 cups cooked whole-wheat pasta
- ¼ cup no-cholesterol mayonnaise
- ½ cup diced celery
- ½ cup diced red bell pepper
- Salt and pepper to taste

Combine all ingredients in a bowl. Cover and refrigerate at least 6 hours.

Waldorf Tuna Salad
Solution Diet, Day 2

    8 ounces canned white tuna, packed in water
    ¼ cup no-cholesterol mayonnaise
    ½ small red apple, cored and chopped
    ½ cup chopped celery
    ¼ cup English walnut pieces

Combine all ingredients. Cover and refrigerate 2 hours.

Conclusion

I began this book with the statement that vital journeys in life often start with the intense desire to help someone you love. So it has been with the writing of this book.

My crusade to understand these diseases, and to help the people who suffer from them, began in response to a plea from my sister, as her expensive, toxic medications failed to stop the progression of her debilitating disease. My efforts in the laboratory were fueled by my son's asthma, which regularly took him to the hospital during the second and third years of his life, while I watched helplessly.

But the impetus to write this book—to share what I know about inflammatory disease, and to put tools to help into the hands of those who need them—came from another quarter. Six years ago, I lost my father to cancer. A week before he died, this simple man, a farmer from the foothills of North Carolina, handed me a sheet of paper, which he called a manifesto for my life. In this powerful document, he charged me with a tremendous responsibility: to use all of my gifts and the resources available to me to fight against major disease.

I have written this book in response to my father's call to arms.

Inflammatory disease is the corruption of one of the body's most elegant systems, and the devastation that this disease wages on the bodies of those afflicted can only be described as tragic. If you've read this book, chances are good that you, or someone you love, suffer from one of these diseases. You're certainly not alone: almost 50 percent of Americans do. And the very category of inflammatory disease—an umbrella that casts shade over conditions as disparate as asthma, allergies, lupus, diabetes, heart disease, and arthritis—continues to expand as our scientific knowledge grows. We are clearly facing a true public health crisis, and inflammation is at the root of this epidemic, as it is at the root of so many diseases.

There has been a push toward understanding the genetic components of these diseases—an understandable push, because there is certainly a genetic component driving this pandemic. But we can no longer ignore the environmental forces—our own behaviors—and the significant role they play. These are the items that we can immediately change, the things that will have immediate impact on our lives and this epidemic.

We are, in a very real sense, the victims of our own affluence. Industrialization has fundamentally altered the sources of our food supply and the balance of nutrients in our diets. Genetically, our bodies are the same as they were fifty thousand years ago, but the foods that we are eating are dramatically different. For example, certain fats, the focus of this book, control the production of inflammatory messengers; others suppress that production. Because of the changes in our food supply, we are eating too many of the fats that increase inflammatory messengers with the resulting diseases, and not enough of the fats that preserve normal immunity.

Unfortunately, these changes have had a radical impact on our bodies: there is a mutiny on the ship, infighting in the ranks, a civil war declared. Our bodies have turned against themselves. It is essential that we now heed the wake-up call, and pull our diets back into balance—and not just because of the threat of inflammatory disease. In fact, some of the very same shifts behind the epidemic in inflammatory disease are the impetus behind another public health crisis of epidemic proportion: obesity.

The picture I have just painted is a sobering one, but you hold part of the solution in your hands. It is possible to reverse the damage done by this dietary imbalance, and I believe that the safe, all-natural, easy-to-follow dietary solution proposed in this book can help.

The Chilton Program is considerably more specific than any other diet currently in the marketplace about the ways our macronutrient choices—the protein, fat, and carbohydrates we eat—impact our health.

In the process of researching this refinement, some apple carts were over-turned. A "bad" omega-6 fatty acid has been found to have extremely po-tent anti-inflammatory potential. Additionally, some of the foods previously thought to be best for us turned out to be loaded with another, very dangerous omega-6.

And, unlike other dietary "solutions," this one is scientifically based. It interrupts the same "billion-dollar pathway" behind bestselling anti-inflammatory medications like Celebrex and Singulair. There is even evidence that it works *more* efficiently than those medications, by disarm-ing the body's ability to make too many of the inflammatory messengers that cause the symptoms and signs of these pernicious diseases.

It is my great hope that I have satisfactorily answered my father's call to arms with the program in this book, which is called the Chilton Pro-gram in honor of him, not myself. I believe that the Chilton Program of-fers a new and revolutionary solution to help those who suffer from inflammatory disease in Western countries to manage their devastating conditions. And I believe that the principles of this program, and the tools within it, can restore our natural balance, so that the affluence of an Inflammation Nation is once again a blessing, and not a curse.

Glossary

acute: a term used to describe a disease of short duration that starts quickly and has severe symptoms

allergy: an acquired, abnormal, and inappropriate immune system response to a substance

antibody: a specialized protein designed to attack bacteria, viruses, and toxic proteins

arachidonic acid (AA): an inflammatory omega-6 fatty acid

autoimmune response: an immune response that takes place against the body's own tissues

B lymphocyte: a type of white blood cell

chronic: long-lasting and recurrent

dihomogammalinolenic acid (DGLA): an anti-inflammatory omega-6 fatty acid

docosahexaenoic acid (DHA): a beneficial omega-3 fatty acid

echium: plant from which stearidonic acid (SDA) is derived

eicosapentaenoic acid (EPA): beneficial omega-3 fatty acid, which blocks the conversion of GLA to AA

enzyme: a protein that causes or speeds up a chemical reaction

essential fatty acids: fatty acids that the body cannot produce; these must be obtained from food

fatty acid: a compound that comes from the breakdown of fat

gammalinolenic acid (GLA): the precursor to the anti-inflammatory dihomogammalinolenic acid

immune system: the body's defense against disease, infection, and foreign substances

institutional review board (IRB): a committee that oversees research done on human subjects

leukotriene: an inflammatory messenger that has many functions, including controlling parts of the inflammatory response

linoleic acid (LA): an omega-6 fatty acid that is extremely prevalent in Western diets

(alpha)linolenic acid (LNA): an omega-3 fatty acid found predominantly in marine plants

lymphocyte: a group of white blood cells

macrophage: a type of white blood cell

metabolic kitchen: a carefully controlled kitchen that prepares meals for subjects in research studies

metabolites: the products of metabolism

neutrophil: a type of white blood cell

NSAID: nonsteroidal anti-inflammatory drug, like aspirin, ibuprofen, and Celebrex

omega-3: a type of polyunsaturated fatty acid that has a double bond three carbons from the end of the fatty acid

omega-6: a type of polyunsaturated fatty acid that has a double bond six carbons from the end of the fatty acid

platelet stickiness: a tendency of platelets, a blood component, to clot

prostaglandin: an inflammatory messenger that has many functions, including controlling parts of the inflammatory response

salicylic acid: the active ingredient in aspirin

stearidonic acid (SDA): an omega-3 fatty acid derived from a plant, with many of the same anti-inflammatory effects as DGLA

steroid (also corticosteroid): a class of medications that reduce swelling and inflammation

T lymphocyte: a type of white blood cell; also called T cell

A LETTER TO YOUR DOCTOR

Dear Doctor,

Currently, one-third to one-half of the citizens in developed countries such as the United States suffer from inflammatory diseases such as asthma, arthritis, allergies, diabetes, lupus, Crohn's disease, eczema, or heart disease, and the incidence of most of these diseases has doubled over the past decade. These disturbing trends have created a generation of sufferers who are desperately seeking an answer to what has caused this epidemic of epidemics, and for new ways to manage their debilitating inflammatory diseases.

For over fifty years, certain fatty acids have been recognized as molecules that serve as critical lipid messengers to healthy organs and tissues, especially one in particular: arachidonic acid (AA). When overproduced, messengers from the metabolism of AA can cause severe, chronic inflammatory diseases. Importantly, inhibition of these messengers is a proven approach for the treatment of inflammatory diseases. This is evidenced by the fact that a Nobel Prize in Medicine was awarded in 1982 for work in elucidating the pathological effects, pathways, and metabolites of AA, and by the blockbuster drugs including aspirin, ibuprofen, Celebrex, Singulair, and Accolate that have resulted from work in this area.

My expertise is in understanding how this dysfunctional AA metabolism in the human body causes disease. Through twenty years of research at the Johns Hopkins and Wake Forest schools of medicine, I developed a discovery platform called Functional Liponomics, which explores causal relationships between specific genes and fatty acids and their effects on human diseases, in order to identify critical points in fatty acid metabolism that lead to human diseases. This technology has generated and/or been used to develop anti-inflammatory dietary strategies that are the subject of forty issued and twenty-nine pending U.S. and foreign patents. More important, this platform has enabled me to design a dietary program (outlined in this book) to manage and control inflammatory messengers that impact a wide range of human diseases.

These strategies are backed by six clinical trials leading to six peer-reviewed publications (see the clinical trial at the end of this book) that were carried out by my laboratory in collaboration with General Clinical Research Centers at major medical centers. Collectively, the studies reveal that the fatty acids that we take into our diets play a critically important role in determining the quantities of inflammatory messengers that we humans produce.

In essence, this program provides foods that are largely devoid of arachidonic acid and are enriched in fatty acids that block inflammatory messenger formation when provided in combination with one another. More specifically, this blend of fatty acids is clinically proven to safely and effectively block the production of leukotrienes and prostaglandins, substances known to cause inflammatory diseases in humans.

The Chilton Program works by utilizing three distinct steps. The initial step is to take as much dietary AA as possible out of the diet. The scientific evidence is unequivocal that reducing dietary AA inhibits the production of inflammatory messengers, and a recent study in the *New England Journal of Medicine* shows that certain subgroups of patients with atherosclerosis and related heart disease are made much worse if these patients eat foods that contain high levels of dietary AA. The second step is to include fatty acids in the diet that will inhibit AA metabolism. Certainly the rationale of this approach is proven, given the success of nonsteroidal anti-inflammatory drugs (NSAIDs). The third step is to maintain the anti-inflammatory benefits gained by my program by eating carbohydrates that maintain stable blood insulin levels. Altering insulin levels exacerbates inflammation, at least in part, by affecting AA metabolism.

My program was designed for the long-term dietary management of inflammatory diseases, and I hope you will consider recommending it to your patients as such. Given its mechanism of action, it is a maintenance system and not a rescue solution. I know that physicians treating patients with inflammatory diseases desperately want to prevent disease flares before they happen, which is why there is such an emphasis in the pharmaceutical industry on maintenance drugs. For example, in a disease such as asthma, it is estimated that almost 70 percent of prescriptions are for maintenance drugs, not rescue medications. Similarly, I believe that for any diet program to affect the long-term improvement of a disease, it must be viewed as a maintenance or management program and not a rescue solution. It is very important to point out that *my program is not intended to replace medications.* It is designed to work synergistically with other medications.

How will you, as a physician, know the program is working for your patients? I have worked closely with a commercial laboratory called Biotechnics, Inc., to develop two reliable tests that measure key polyunsaturated fatty acids such as AA and eicosapentaenoic acid (EPA) in blood and leukotriene levels in urine. I believe that results from these tests will become widely used indicators of inflammation in the future. The instructions for these tests and the address for Biotechnics, Inc., are included in chapter 10 of this book, and are also found at www.inflammationnation.com. Consequently, changes in the blood fatty acids and inflammatory messengers produced in your patients can be monitored weekly or monthly to assure that my program is having its intended anti-inflammatory effects.

For decades, physicians have been looking for safe and effective dietary solutions for their patients who suffer from chronic inflammatory diseases. Based on the best science available, I believe that I have designed a powerful dietary program that a physician can use, together with anti-inflammatory drugs, to combat inflammation.

I am incredibly excited to have the opportunity to help the millions of people who suffer from the devastating epidemic of inflammatory diseases. I also look forward to building strong partnerships with physicians such as yourself, in order to improve the quality of life of your patients. Your input and comments are always welcome, and I will use them to improve the current program.

Warmest regards,
Floyd H. "Ski" Chilton III, Ph.D.

Inflammatory Index=([AA]/[AA]+[EPA]) ([AA])(EPA concentration factor or ECF)

EPA Concentration Factor (ECF) Values

1,000 mg of EPA per 100 g portion = 0.1

500 mg to 1,000 mg of EPA per 100 g portion = 0.2

250 mg to 500 mg of EPA per 100 g portion = 0.4

100 mg to 250 mg of EPA per 100 g portion = 0.6

1 to 100 mg of EPA per 100 g portion = 0.8

0 mg of EPA per 100 g portion = 1.0

Appendix B

Human Nutrition and Metabolism

Addition of Eicosapentaenoic Acid to γ-Linolenic Acid–Supplemented Diets Prevents Serum Arachidonic Acid Accumulation in Humans[1]

J. Brooke Barham,* Michelle B. Edens,* Alfred N. Fonteh,* Margaret M. Johnson,[†]
Linda Easter** and Floyd H. Chilton*[‡][††][2]

*Departments of *Internal Medicine (Section on Pulmonary and Critical Care Medicine), ‡Biochemistry and ††Physiology/Pharmacology, and **General Clinical Research Center Wake Forest University School of Medicine, Winston-Salem, NC 27157 and †Department of Medicine, Mayo Clinic Jacksonville, Jacksonville, FL 32224*

ABSTRACT   Previous studies reveal that supplementation of human diets with γ-linolenic acid (GLA) reduces the generation of lipid mediators of inflammation and attenuates clinical symptoms of chronic inflammatory disorders such as rheumatoid arthritis. However, we have shown that supplementation with this same fatty acid also causes a marked increase in serum arachidonate (AA) levels, a potentially harmful side effect. The objective of this study was to design a supplementation strategy that maintained the capacity of GLA to reduce lipid mediators without causing elevations in serum AA levels. Initial in vitro studies utilizing HEP-G2 liver cells revealed that addition of eicosapentaenoic acid (EPA) blocked Δ-5-desaturase activity, the terminal enzymatic step in AA synthesis. To test the in vivo effects of a GLA and EPA combination in humans, adult volunteers consuming controlled diets supplemented these diets with 3.0 g/d of GLA and EPA. This supplementation strategy significantly increased serum levels of EPA, but did not increase AA levels. EPA and the elongation product of GLA, dihomo-γ-linolenic acid (DGLA) levels in neutrophil glycerolipids increased significantly during the 3-wk supplementation period. Neutrophils isolated from volunteers fed diets supplemented with GLA and EPA released similar quantities of AA, but synthesized significantly lower quantities of leukotrienes compared with their neutrophils before supplementation. This study revealed that a GLA and EPA supplement combination may be utilized to reduce the synthesis of proinflammatory AA metabolites, and importantly, not induce potentially harmful increases in serum AA levels.   J. Nutr. 130: 1925–1931, 2000.

KEY WORDS: • arachidonic acid • γ-linolenic acid • inflammation • leukotrienes • neutrophils • humans

γ-Linolenic acid (GLA)[3] is an 18-carbon polyunsaturated fatty acid of the (n-6) series. When given as a dietary supplement, this fatty acid has been shown to relieve the signs and symptoms of chronic inflammatory diseases, including rheumatoid arthritis and atopic dermatitis (Andreassi et al. 1997, Kunkel et al. 1981, Leventhal et al. 1993 and 1994, Lovell et al. 1981, Morse et al. 1989, Tate et al. 1989, Zurier et al. 1996). Many of the clinical effects of GLA supplementation have been attributed to its capacity to block the metabolism of arachidonic acid (AA) to bioactive eicosanoids. However, this is a somewhat paradoxical finding because GLA, via its metabolism by elongase and Δ-5-desaturase activities, is a poten-

tial precursor of AA; thus, adding dietary GLA might be expected to increase AA levels with subsequent proinflammatory effects. Recent in vitro and in vivo studies have begun to resolve this paradox by demonstrating that inflammatory cells such as human neutrophils contain the elongase but not the Δ-5-desaturase activity, and thus dietary GLA supplementation leads to the accumulation of dihomo-γ-linolenic acid (DGLA) and not AA in cellular glycerolipids. Importantly, neutrophils from subjects supplemented with GLA produce less leukotriene B₄ (LTB₄) than they did before supplementation (Johnson et al. 1997, Ziboh and Fletcher 1992). Together, these studies reveal that the endogenous elongase activity in certain inflammatory cells can be utilized to synthesize close structural analogs of AA (i.e., DGLA) from appropriate dietary precursors, and these analogs may then affect AA metabolism (Chilton-Lopez et al. 1996, Johnson et al. 1997).

In contrast to neutrophils, GLA supplementation can markedly increase serum AA, suggesting that dietary GLA in circulation has the potential to be both elongated to DGLA and subsequently desaturated to AA. Thus, in vivo GLA supplementation in humans attenuates AA metabolism in certain inflammatory cells such as neutrophils, but can also

[1] Supported by National Institutes of Health Grants RO1 AI 24985, RO1 AI 42022, and Wake Forest University School of Medicine General Clinic Research Center with Grant M01-RR07122.
[2] To whom correspondence should be addressed.
[3] Abbreviations used: AA, arachidonic acid; DGLA, dihomo-γ-linolenic acid; DMEM, Dulbecco's modified Eagle's medium; EPA, eicospentaenoic acid; GCRC, General Clinical Research Center; GLA, γ-linolenic acid; HBSS, Hanks' balanced salt solution; oleic acid; LA, linoleic acid; LTB₄, leukotriene B₄; NICI-GC/MS, negative ion chemical ionization-gas chromatography/mass spectrometry; OA, xxxxx; 20-OH, 20-hydroxy; PGB₂, prostaglandin B₂.

0022-3166/00 $3.00 © 2000 American Society for Nutritional Sciences.
Manuscript received 27 August 1999. Initial review completed 29 September 1999. Revision accepted 21 March 2000.

Note: Reprinted from *Journal of Nutrition*, vol. 130, no. 8, August 2000.

BARHAM ET AL.

TABLE 1

Nutritional composition of the controlled diet[1]

Nutrient	d 1	d 2	d 3	d 4	d 5	Mean
Protein, % total energy	21.08	20.44	19.22	18.71	19.56	19.71
Carbohydrate, % total energy	55.73	55.73	56.35	57.79	56.74	56.46
Fat, % total energy	25.95	26.11	26.06	25.56	26.55	26.05
Cholesterol, mg/d	201.45	503.98	198.99	285.40	251.58	288.28
Total SFA, g/d	22.91	15.27	18.71	13.75	16.72	17.47
Total PUFA, g/d	12.89	16.82	10.40	15.42	15.15	14.14
Total MUFA, g/d	17.49	21.67	20.91	22.09	23.33	21.10
Linoleic acid, g/d	11.17	14.91	9.33	14.38	13.34	12.63
Linolenic acid, g/d	1.63	1.34	0.95	0.78	1.44	1.23

[1] Abbreviations: SFA, saturated fatty acid; PUFA, polyunsaturated fatty acid; MUFA, monounsaturated fatty acid.

lead to the potentially adverse effect of increasing serum AA levels. Previous studies have suggested that the accumulation of AA in serum can have important consequences in humans. For example, AA has been shown to enhance the formation of platelet-aggregating endoperoxides and thromboxanes (Hamberg et al. 1974 and 1975, Smith et al. 1974, Willis 1974). Moreover, high levels of AA in humans result in an increased tendency for the secondary irreversible phase of platelet aggregation (Seyberth et al. 1975). In most cases, an increase in sensitivity of platelets to aggregating stimuli is not desirable.

The observation that serum AA accumulates after GLA supplementation raises important concerns about the long-term effect of this dietary supplementation strategy (Johnson et al.1997). It also highlights the need to find dietary strategies that will produce natural inhibitors (such as DGLA) of AA within inflammatory cells, thereby reducing the synthesis of proinflammatory eicosanoids without increasing serum levels of AA. We tested the hypothesis that the addition of the (n-3) fatty acid product of the Δ-5-desaturase reaction, eicosapentaenoic acid (EPA), attenuates the in vitro and in vivo conversion of DGLA to AA by nonneutrophil sources, thereby reducing serum AA accumulation observed during GLA supplementation.

SUBJECTS AND METHODS

Materials. Prostaglandin B_2 (PGB_2), octadeuterated arachidonic acid and trideuterated stearic acid were obtained from Biomol Research Laboratories (Plymouth Meeting, MA). Leukotriene B_4 (LTB_4), 20-hydroxy-LTB_4 (20-OH-LTB_4) and all fatty acids (GLA, linoleic acid [LA], oleic acid [OA], DGLA, AA and EPA) were obtained from Cayman Chemical (Rockford, IL). Ficoll-Paque was obtained from Pharmacia (Uppsala, Sweden). Dextran 70 (6g/L) in 0.9g/L sodium chloride was purchased from Abbott Laboratories (North Chicago, IL). Bakerbond solid phase extraction octadecyl (C_{18}) disposable columns were obtained from J. T. Baker Chemical (Phillipsburg, NJ). Ionophore A23187 was purchased from Calbiochem (San Diego, CA). All solvents (HPLC grade) were obtained from Fisher Scientific (Norcross, GA). Hanks' balanced salt solution (HBSS) with and without calcium was purchased from Mediatech Cellgro (Herndon, VA). Pentafluorobenzyl bromide (20 mL/L in acetonitrile) and diisopropyl ethylamine (20 mL/L in acetonitrile) were obtained from Pierce (Rockford, IL). Dulbecco's modified Eagle's medium (DMEM), insulin-transferrin-selenium-X and fetal bovine serum were purchased from Life Technologies (Grand Island, NY). The penicillin + streptomycin mixture was obtained from Bio Whittaker (Walkersville, MD). BIO-EFA borage oil capsules were a generous gift from Health From the Sun (Sunapee, NH). Twin EPA extra-strength fish oil concentrate capsules were obtained from Twin Laboratories (Ronkonkoma, NY).

Dietary protocols. The protocols used were approved by the Institutional Review Board and written consent was obtained from each volunteer before starting the study. Healthy volunteers had baseline interviews with a nutritionist for diet history and a review of study procedures. Height, weight, activity levels and usual eating habits were assessed to determine energy needs and to eliminate potentially noncompliant subjects. Energy intake needs were established using the Harris Benedict equation with the addition of a factor of 1.3–1.7 for activity level. All food consumed by subjects for the 21-d outpatient period was prepared by the Metabolic Kitchen of the Wake Forest University School of Medicine General Clinical Research Center (GCRC) using a 5-d menu cycle prepared under controlled, constant conditions. The nutritional composition of the diet is given in **Table 1**. Subjects reported to the GCRC five times per week to be weighed and receive their meals. Subjects received daily checklists of foods to be consumed and returned them with notations of any deviations from the diet provided. Regular contact and communication with the GCRC nutritionists were maintained, and minor modifications to the menus were made as needed to ensure compliance. Weights were monitored and energy intakes adjusted (in increments of 418 kJ) if a weight change of >1 kg from baseline was observed for three consecutive visits or total weight change exceeded 1.5 kg. All subjects maintained body weight within 1.5 kg of baseline weight during the study as seen in **Table 2**; only one subject required adjustment of energy intake during the study (Table 2). **Table 3** shows the composition of several minor fatty acids consumed during the 5-d menu cycle as determined by negative ion chemical ionization gas chromatography/mass spectrometry (NICI-GC/MS; see below). There were no adverse effects reported by any of the volunteers.

TABLE 2

Subject data

Subject	Baseline weight	Baseline BMI[1]	Energy intake	Final weight
	kg	kg/m²	kJ/d	kg
1	84.17	24.0	12,970	84.17
2	69.21	25.0	10,042	68.36
3	68.48	22.6	8786	67.36
4	62.86	24.2	10,460	62.91
5	65.94	25.8	9205	65.91
6	80.45	23.8	12,134	79.27
7	82.00	25.9	12,552	82.54
8	52.52	20.5	8368	53.54
9	56.42	24.7	7113	55.45
10	57.96	19.6	10,042	57.64
11	81.18	23.3	11,297	81.09
12	53.24	21.0	7950	54.72

[1] BMI, body mass index.

TABLE 3

The fatty acid composition of the 5-d rotating menu[1,2]

	AA	EPA	DGLA	GLA
		mg		
d 1	49.7	3.1	18.4	45.8
d 2	53.6	16.6	15.7	35.2
d 3	92.2	3.5	23.5	37.4
d 4	51.8	1.0	10.6	35.1
d 5	59.2	6.8	16.8	31.6

[1] The total amount of food for a 42-y-old male was combined and homogenized. Lipids were extracted, hydrolyzed and quantities of fatty acids were determined by negative ion chemical ionization-gas chromatography/mass spectrometry as described in Subjects and Methods. These data are the total fatty acids (mg) for a 5-d rotating menu.
[2] Abbreviations: AA, arachidonic acid; EPA, eicosapentaenoic acid; DGLA, dihomo-γ-linolenic acid; GLA, γ-linolenic acid.

Protocol A. Healthy volunteers (n = 4; 2 men and 2 women; ages ranging from 25 to 37 y) consumed the controlled diet (described above). They took 10 capsules (5 capsules in the morning and 5 capsules in the evening) of borage oil (BIO-EFA) containing ~3.0 g GLA/d. Blood was obtained, and serum and neutrophils were isolated after an overnight fast, the morning before starting the supplementation and each week of the supplementation.

Protocol B. Healthy volunteers (n = 12; 5 women and 7 men; ages ranging from 23 to 42 y) consumed the controlled diet (described above) and were supplemented with oils enriched in GLA (~3 g/d) and EPA (~3 g/d). Specifically, they consumed 10 capsules/d (5 capsules in the morning and 5 capsules at night) of BIO-EFA and 5 capsules/d (3 capsules in the morning and 2 capsules at night) of concentrated fish oil (Twin EPA), for 21 d. NICI-GC/MS (see below) revealed that the Twin EPA capsule contained ~600 mg of EPA and ~280 mg of docosahexaenoic acid (DHA). Blood was obtained, and serum and neutrophils isolated after an overnight fast, the morning before supplementation, each week during the supplementation and 2 wk after ending the supplementation (washout).

Analysis of serum lipids. Venous blood (~2 mL) was taken from each volunteer at each time point described above, and serum was isolated as previously described (Chilton et al. 1993). The lipids from a 100-μL aliquot of the serum were extracted by the method of Bligh and Dyer (1959). Trideuterated stearic acid (100 ng) and octadeuterated arachidonic acid (100 ng) were added as internal standards to the samples. Fatty acids were cleaved from glycerolipids by base hydrolysis [0.5 mol/L potassium hydroxide in methanol/water (3:1) for 30 min at 60°C]. Reactions were stopped by neutralizing the mixture using 0.5 mL of 6 mol/L HCl. Samples were then loaded onto Bakerbond octadecyl columns and fatty acid–enriched fractions were extracted as previously described (Chilton et al. 1993). Fatty acids were then converted to pentafluorobenzyl esters using 20% pentafluorobenzyl bromide and 20% diisopropylethylamine for 30 min at 40°C. Quantities of fatty acids were then determined by NICI-GC/MS as described below.

Analysis of fatty acid composition of neutrophil glycerolipids. Neutrophils were isolated from whole blood of each volunteer at each time point and were suspended at 10×10^9 cells/L in HBSS containing calcium. Mole quantities of fatty acids were determined as previously described (Chilton et al. 1993). Briefly, total lipids were extracted by the method of Bligh and Dyer (1959). Octadeuterated arachidonic acid and trideuterated stearic acid (100 ng each) were added to samples as internal standards. Fatty acids were hydrolyzed from glycerolipids utilizing base hydrolysis, and fatty acids extracted and derivatized as described above. Quantities of fatty acids were then determined by NICI-GC/MS as described below.

Analysis of products after neutrophil stimulation. Isolated neutrophils were suspended in HBSS containing calcium at a concentration of 10×10^9 cells/L. Neutrophils were then stimulated by the addition of ionophore A23187 (1 μmol/L) and reactions allowed to proceed for 5 min. When analyzing the capacity of neutrophils to release fatty acids, reactions were terminated with methanol/chloroform (2:1, v/v). Trideuterated stearic acid (100 ng) and octadeuterated arachidonic (100 ng) acid were added as internal standards. Mole quantities of fatty acids released were determined utilizing NICI-GC/MS as described below. When analyzing the capacity of neutrophils to synthesize leukotrienes, reactions were terminated by removing cells from supernatant fluids utilizing centrifugation (400 × g, 5 min, 4°C). Supernatant fluids were removed and acidified with 9% formic acid. PGB₂ (250 ng) was added to each sample as an internal standard before the fatty acids and eicosanoids were extracted with four volumes of ethyl acetate (2X). This extract was then loaded onto an LC-18 reverse-phase narrowbore HPLC column (25 cm × 2.1 mm) purchased from Supelco (Bellefonte, PA); the leukotrienes were eluted with a mobile phase of methanol/water/phosphoric acid (55:45:0.02, v/v/v, pH 5.6) at a flow rate of 0.3 mL/min. After 5 min, the methanol composition of the mobile phase was increased to 100% over 30 min. The areas under the UV peaks (at 270 nm) corresponding to LTB₄, LTB₅, 6-*trans* isomers and 20-OH-LTB₄ were identified and compared with the peak area of PGB₂ that was added as an internal standard. Mole quantities of leukotrienes were determined utilizing standard curves.

Analysis of the fatty acid composition of the food samples from the 5-d rotating menu. A total day's food from each day of the menu cycle was homogenized using a blender. Lipids were extracted from the 5-d liquefied preparation by the method of Bligh and Dyer (1959). Octadeuterated arachidonic acid (100 ng) and trideuterated stearic acid (100 ng) were added as internal standards. Fatty acids were hydrolyzed from glycerolipids by base hydrolysis, extracted and derivatized as described above. Quantities of fatty acids were determined by NICI-GC/MS as described below.

Analysis of the fatty acid composition of borage oil and fish oil capsules. The contents of the capsules were suspended in methanol/chloroform (1:1, v/v). Octadeuterated arachidonic acid and trideuterated stearic acid (100 ng each) were added as internal standards. Fatty acids were hydrolyzed from glycerolipids by base hydrolysis, and fatty acids extracted and derivatized as described above. Mole quantities of fatty acids were determined by NICI-GC/MS.

In vitro fatty acid metabolism in HEP-G2 cells. HEP-G2 cells (10^6) were cultured in 6 mL of DMEM culture medium supplemented with 1 mL/L penicillin + streptomycin, 1 mL/L fetal bovine serum and 1 mL/L insulin + transferrin at 37°C in 5% CO₂. Solvents were removed from EPA and DGLA under a stream of nitrogen, and these fatty acids were resuspended in DMEM containing 1% fetal bovine serum. This buffer solution was incubated with HEP-G2 cells for 24 h at fatty acids concentrations ranging from 0 to 50 μmol/L. After 24 h, the media were removed and adherent cells washed (2X) with HBSS containing human serum albumin (0.25g/L). HEP-G2 cells were then removed (rubber policeman) from flasks and suspended in HBSS/methanol/chloroform (1:2:1, v/v/v). Lipids were extracted by the method of Bligh and Dyer (1959) as described above. Octadeuterated arachidonic acid (100 ng) and trideuterated stearic acid (100 ng) were added as internal standards. Fatty acids were removed from glycerolipids by base hydrolysis, and fatty acids extracted and derivatized as described above. Quantities of fatty acids were determined by NICI-GC/MS.

Negative ion chemical ionization-gas chromatography/mass spectrometry (NICI-GC/MS). NICI-GC/MS analysis was conducted on a single-stage quadropole mass spectrometer (Hewlett-Packard 5989; Greensboro, NC) as previously described (Chilton et al. 1993). The gas chromatography was performed on a Hewlett-Packard 5890 GC using a 30-m DB-17 fused silica column (SPB-5; 0.25-mm film thickness; Supelco). The initial column temperature was 60°C. The column was heated to 220°C at a rate of 40°C/min with a subsequent increase in temperature to 280°C at a rate of 5°C/min. The injector temperature was maintained at 250°C. Each injection was performed in the splitless mode. A volume of 1 μL from 200 μL of recovered material dissolved in hexane was injected. Helium was used as a carrier gas. The pentafluorobenzyl esters were analyzed using selected ion-recording techniques to monitor GLA (*m/z* 277), LA (*m/z* 279), OA (*m/z* 281), EPA (*m/z* 301), DGLA (*m/z* 305), AA (*m/z* 303), trideuterated stearic acid (*m/z* 286) and octadeuterioarachidonate

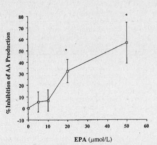

FIGURE 1 Percentage inhibition of arachidonic acid (AA) production induced by eicosapentaenoic acid (EPA) addition in HEP-G2 cells. HEP-G2 cells were maintained in culture supplemented with 20 μmol/L dihomo-γ-linolenic acid (DGLA) and varying concentrations of EPA. After 24 h, cellular AA was determined by negative ion chemical ionization-gas chromatography/mass spectrometry (NICI-GC/MS) as described in Subjects and Methods. These data are expressed as the percentage inhibition of AA biosynthesis by EPA and are means $\pm$ SEM, $n = 4$. *$P \leq 0.05$ vs. 0 μmol/L. Regression equation: $y = 1.9170 + 36.808x$, $r^2 = 0.993$.

(m/z 311). A standard mixture of the aforementioned fatty acids was injected and analyzed by NICI-GC/MS before each biological sample to obtain precise retention times.

Data analysis. The data are presented as means $\pm$ SEM or as percentages of baseline values (LTB$_4$ production and influence of EPA on HEP-G2 cells). Differences were tested for significance ($P < 0.05$) using a Student's t test for paired samples.

RESULTS

Influence of EPA on Δ-5-desaturase activity in HEP-G2 cells. Initial experiments in this study examined whether EPA, a Δ-5-desaturase product, could inhibit the conversion of DGLA to AA in a human hepatocarcinoma cell line, HEP-G2. These HEP-G2 cells exhibit morphological features of mature hepatocytes (Aden et al. 1979). Moreover, this cell line is a relevant experimental model for investigating fatty acid metabolism of the human liver (Angeletti and Tacconi de Alaniz 1995). The addition of DGLA to HEP-G2 cells resulted in the conversion of DGLA to AA. For example, addition of 20 μmol/L DGLA to the HEP-G2 cells markedly increased cellular AA levels. Concomitant addition of EPA with a constant amount of DGLA caused a dose-dependent attenuation in the conversion of DGLA to AA (**Fig. 1**). EPA at 50 μmol/L inhibited AA formation from DGLA (20 μmol/L) by 50%. These data demonstrate the capacity of EPA to block Δ-5-desaturase activity in isolated hepatocytes.

Influence of the combination of GLA and EPA on the fatty acid compositions of serum lipids. A concern with long-term GLA supplementation is that a marked increase in serum levels of AA may occur. Therefore, dietary strategies that allow the accumulation of potential inhibitors of AA metabolism without increasing serum AA would be valuable. Because EPA inhibited Δ-5-desaturase in HEP-G2 cells, we determined whether EPA could similarly suppress hepatic conversion of DGLA to AA in humans. Two groups of volunteers consumed control diets (see Subjects and Methods) and were supplemented with either GLA (3.0 g/d) alone or a combination of GLA (3.0 g/d) and EPA (3.0 g/d). **Figure 2** (*upper panel*) illustrates that GLA alone markedly increased

serum AA and DGLA levels within 3 wk of the initiation of GLA ingestion. In contrast, the combination of EPA with GLA did not increase serum AA levels (Fig. 2, *low panel*), suggesting that it is possible to block Δ-5-desaturase in humans with EPA. However, the GLA and EPA combination markedly increased serum EPA levels. After a 2-wk washout period, EPA levels returned to baseline levels. A previous study in our laboratory demonstrated that AA and DGLA levels increase in response to GLA supplementation and return to baseline values after 2 wk (Johnson et al. 1997). Together, these data suggest that the addition of EPA to human diets containing high levels of GLA provides a means to block increases in serum AA.

Influence of the combination of GLA and EPA on the fatty acid composition of human neutrophils. When subjects were supplemented with a GLA and EPA combination, both DGLA and EPA were significantly increased at wk 3 compared with the baseline values (**Fig. 3**). AA levels in neutrophil lipids did not change. GLA supplementation alone did not increase AA or EPA levels in neutrophil glycerolipids (not shown), but did result in an increase in DGLA levels from 0.15 $\pm$ 0.02 to 0.27 $\pm$ 0.03 nmol/5 $\times$ 10^6 cells after supplementation.(Johnson et al. 1997). In addition, these data are consistent with previous in vitro observations that show human

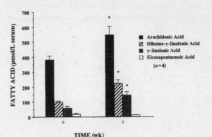

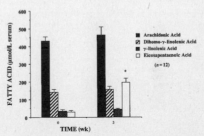

FIGURE 2 Effects of γ-linolenic acid (GLA; *upper panel*) and a combination of GLA and eicospentaenoic acid (EPA) supplementation (*lower panel*) on serum concentrations of fatty acids. Serum fatty acid compositions were determined before (wk 0) or after 3 wk of supplementation by negative ion chemical ionization-gas chromatography/mass spectrometry (NICI-GC/MS). Values are means $\pm$ SEM. *Significantly different from wk 0, $P < 0.05$.

GLA AND EPA SUPPLEMENTATION

1929

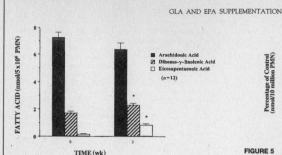

FIGURE 3 Effects of γ-linolenic acid (GLA) and eicospentaenoic acid (EPA) supplementation on the fatty acid composition of glycerolipids in neutrophil membranes. Values are means ± SEM. *Significantly different from wk 0, $P < 0.05$. Abbreviation: PMN, polymorphonuclear leukocytes.

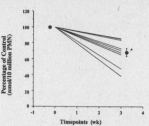

FIGURE 5 Effects of γ-linolenic acid (GLA) and eicospentaenoic acid (EPA) supplementation on the biosynthesis of leukotriene B_4 (LTB_4), 20-hydroxy (20-OH)-LTB_4 and 6-trans-isomers-LTB_4 by A23187-stimulated neutrophils. Neutrophils, isolated before (wk 0) and 3 wk after supplementation were stimulated with 1 μmol/L A23187. The lines represent the percentage of control values for each subject that participated in study and (●) represents the mean ± SEM, $n = 10$. *Significantly different from wk 0, $P < 0.05$. Abbreviation, PMN, polymorphonuclear leukocytes.

neutrophils contain elongase, but lack Δ-5-desaturase activity (Chilton-Lopez et al. 1996).

Influence of the combination of GLA and EPA on the release of fatty acids and the production of LTB_4 and its metabolites by stimulated neutrophils. A final set of experiments was designed to investigate the influence of the GLA + EPA combination on the release of AA and the production of leukotrienes by neutrophils after stimulation with ionophore A23187. **Figure 4** shows the amounts of AA, DGLA and EPA released from stimulated neutrophil glycerolipids at baseline and 3 wk after the GLA + EPA combination. Release of DGLA and EPA from neutrophil glycerolipids was significantly increased after GLA/EPA supplementation. However, the quantity of AA released from neutrophils did not change.

Quantities of LTB_4, 20-OH-LTB_4 and the 6-trans isomers of LTB_4 were determined by HPLC and are expressed as percentage of control in **Figure 5**. There was a significant drop in total leukotriene production from neutrophils 3 wk after

dietary GLA + EPA supplementation. Concomitant with a decrease in leukotrienes of the 4 series, there was an increase in leukotriene B_5 derived from released EPA (**Fig. 6**).

DISCUSSION

Studies by several investigators have demonstrated that dietary supplementation with GLA has the potential to reduce inflammation. This reduction in inflammation has been attributed to the capacity of the elongation product of GLA, DGLA, to block the synthesis of AA products and the capacity of DGLA to be converted to oxidized products that have anti-inflammatory activities (Billah et al. 1985, Chilton-Lopez et al. 1996, DeLuca et al. 1999, Iversen et al. 1991 and 1992, Vanderhoek et al. 1980). Our previous studies (Chilton et al.

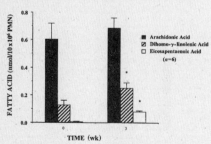

FIGURE 4 Effects of γ-linolenic acid (GLA) and eicospentaenoic acid (EPA) supplementation on the release of fatty acids from glycerolipids of neutrophils stimulated with ionophore A23187. Neutrophils, isolated before (wk 0) and 3 wk after supplementation were stimulated with 1 μmol/L A23187. Values are means ± SEM. *Significantly different from wk 0, $P < 0.05$. Abbreviation: PMN, polymorphonuclear leukocytes.

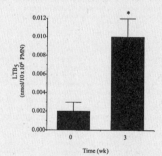

FIGURE 6 Effects of γ-linolenic acid (GLA) and eicospentaenoic acid (EPA) supplementation on the biosynthesis of leukotriene B_5 (LTB_5) by A23187-stimulated neutrophils. Neutrophils were isolated before supplementation (wk 0) and after 3 wk. After supplementation neutrophils were stimulated with 1 μmol/L A23187. Values are means ± SEM, $n = 12$. *Significantly different from wk 0, $P < 0.05$. Abbreviation: PMN, polymorphonuclear leukocytes.

1930   BARHAM ET AL.

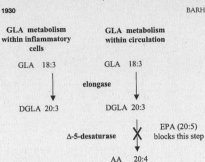

GLA metabolism within inflammatory cells

GLA 18:3

↓

DGLA 20:3

Δ-5-desaturase

AA 20:4

GLA metabolism within circulation

GLA 18:3

elongase ↓

DGLA 20:3

EPA (20:5) blocks this step

FIGURE 7 Mechanism of inhibition of Δ-5-desaturase by dietary eicospentaenoic acid (EPA). Abbreviations: GLA, γ-linolenic acid; DGLA, dihomo-γ-linolenic acid; AA, arachidonic acid.

1993, Chilton-Lopez et al. 1996, Johnson et al.1996) and those of Ziboh and Fletcher (1992) have demonstrated that supplementation of low-to-moderate fat diets with GLA markedly decreases the capacity of inflammatory cells such as human neutrophils to produce leukotrienes (Johnson et al.1997). We further demonstrated that the likely mechanism of inhibition by GLA stems from its capacity to be elongated by an endogenous elongase activity within the neutrophil to a close structural analog of AA, DGLA (**Fig. 7**). However, neutrophils cannot further desaturate DGLA to AA because they lack Δ-5-desaturase activity (Chilton-Lopez et al.1996). Thus, the endogenous elongase activity within inflammatory cells can be utilized to synthesize close structural analogs of AA (i.e., DGLA) from appropriate dietary precursors. It is postulated that these analogs affect AA metabolism, thereby mitigating clinical manifestations induced by AA metabolites.

A potentially important side effect of GLA supplementation is elongation of GLA to DGLA and further desaturation via Δ-5-desaturase to AA by enzymes in the liver. This causes a marked increase in serum AA levels. In a previous study of AA supplementation in humans, similar increases in serum AA levels were associated with an increase in the in vivo aggregation of platelets (Seyberth et al.1975). This increase in platelet sensitivity raised concerns about potentially harmful cardiovascular side effects and the long-term safety of any dietary strategy that increases serum AA levels, including those current formulations being sold in nutraceutical markets.

The current study was designed to determine whether dietary strategies could be designed that have the anti-inflammatory potential of GLA without leading to increases in serum AA. This was accomplished by the addition of the Δ-5-desaturase product of the (n-3) pathway, EPA. Initial in vitro experiments demonstrated that EPA had the capacity to block Δ-5-desaturase activity in an isolated hepatocarcinoma cell line. These experiments were followed by in vivo studies that showed EPA supplementation of human diets prevented the accumulation of serum AA in response to GLA without inhibiting accumulation of DGLA in neutrophils. Thus, both in vivo and in vitro studies revealed that EPA may act as an end product inhibitor of the Δ-5-desaturase.

We further examined the influence of the GLA + EPA combination on leukotriene generation. The capacity of human neutrophils to release AA was not influenced by the GLA + EPA supplementation. In contrast, their capacity to generate leukotrienes (LTB₄, 20-OH-LTB₄ and related isomers) was

inhibited significantly (~40%) compared with neutrophils from these same volunteers before supplementation. The inhibition observed in this study was greater than what has been observed before for EPA alone (Chilton et al.1993). In contrast, the inhibition with EPA/GLA was somewhat less than that seen in a previous study in our laboratory with GLA alone (Johnson et al. 1997). However, the differences in leukotriene generation in these studies were not powered sufficiently to detect statistically significant differences and may be a function of biologic variability among the volunteers.

Clinicians, patients, pharmaceutical and nutraceutical companies are all increasingly utilizing natural products for the treatment of clinical disorders. As this trend continues, it is important that these products be both safe and effective. Overall, little attention has been paid to the potentially adverse effects of dietary supplements and specifically, dietary fatty acid supplementation strategies. This study shows how a potentially important complication, arising from supplementation with a simple fatty acid, can be avoided by using appropriate fatty acid combinations. As the nutraceutical industry continues to experience explosive growth, it will be increasingly important to understand the safety profiles of dietary supplements and avoid complications that arise from such supplements.

ACKNOWLEDGMENTS

The authors would like to express their gratitude to the technicians in the metabolic kitchen of the GCRC for help in the planning and preparation of the participants' controlled diets. We would also like to thank Donald Misch for his support in the preparation of this paper.

LITERATURE CITED

Aden, D. P., Fogel, A., Plotkin, S., Damjanov, I. & Knowles, B. B. (1979) Controlled synthesis of HBsAg in differentiated human liver carcinoma derived cell line. Nature (Lond.) 282: 615–616.

Andreassi, M., Forleo, P., Di Lorio, A., Masci, S., Abate, G. & Amerio, P. (1997) Efficacy of γ-linolenic acid in the treatment of patients with atopic dermatitis. J. Int. Med. Res. 25: 266–274.

Angeletti, C. & Tacconi de Alaniz, M. J. (1995) Fatty acid uptake and metabolism in HEP-G2 human-heptoma cells. Mol. Cell. Biol. 143: 99–105.

Billah, M. M., Bryant, R. R. & Siegel, M. I. (1985) Lipoxygenase products of arachidonic acid modulate the biosynthesis of platelet-activating factor (1–0-alkyl-2-acetyl-sn-glycero-3-phosphocholine) by human neutrophils via phospholipase A₂. J. Biol. Chem. 260: 6899–6906.

Bligh, E. G. & Dyer, W. T. (1959) A rapid method of total lipid extraction and purification. Can. J. Biochem. Physiol. 37: 911–920.

Chilton, F. H., Patel, M., Fonteh, A. N., Hubbard, W. C. & Triggiani, M. (1993) Dietary n-3 fatty acid effects on neutrophil lipid composition and mediator production. Influence on duration and dosage. J. Clin. Investig. 91: 115–122.

Chilton-Lopez, T., Surette, M. E., Swan, D. D., Fonteh, A. N., Johnson, M. M. & Chilton, F. H. (1996) Metabolism of gamma-linoleic acid in human neutrophils. J. Immunol. 156: 291–2947.

DeLuca, P., Rossetti, R. G., Alavian, C., Karim, P. & Zurier, R. B. (1999) Effects of gammalinolenic acid on interleukin-1β and tumor necrosis factor-α secretion by stimulated human peripheral blood monocytes: studies in vitro and in vivo. J. Investig. Med. 47: 246–250.

Hamberg, M., Svenson, J. & Samuelsson, B. (1975) Thromboxanes: a new group of biologically active compounds derived from prostaglandin endoperoxides. Proc. Natl. Acad. Sci. U.S.A. 72: 2994–2998.

Hamberg, M., Svenson, J., Wakabayashi, T. & Samuelsson, B. (1974) Isolation and structure of two prostaglandin endoperoxides that cause platelet aggregation. Proc. Natl. Acad. Sci. U.S.A. 71: 345–349.

Iversen, L., Fogh, K., Bojesen, G. & Kragballe, K. (1991) Linoleic acid and dihomogammalinolenic acid inhibit leukotriene B₄ formation and stimulate the formation of their 15-lipoxygenase products by human neutrophils in vitro. Evidence of formation of antiinflammatory compounds. Agents Actions 33: 286–291.

Iversen, L., Fogh, K. & Kragballe, K. (1992) Effect of dihomogammalinolenic acid and its 15-lipoxygenase metabolite on eicosanoid metabolism by human mononuclear leukocytes in vitro: selective inhibition of the 5-lipoxygenase pathway. Arch. Dermatol. Res. 284: 222–226.

Johnson, M. M., Swan, D. D., Surette, M. E., Stegner, J., Chilton, T., Fonteh, A. N. & Chilton, F. H. (1997) Dietary supplementation with γ-linolenic acid alters

GLA AND EPA SUPPLEMENTATION   **1931**

fatty acid content and eicosanoid production in healthy humans. J. Nutr. 127: 1435–1444.

Kunkel, S. L., Ogawa, H., Ward, P. A. & Zuner, R. B. (1981) Suppression of chronic inflammation by evening primrose. Prog. Lipid Res. 20: 885–888.

Leventhal, L. J., Boyce, E. G. & Zurier, R. B. (1993) Treatment of rheumatoid arthritis with gammalinolenic acid. Ann. Intern. Med. 119: 867–873.

Leventhal, L. J., Boyce, E. G. & Zurier, R. B. (1994) Treatment of rheumatoid arthritis with blackcurrant seed oil. Br. J. Rheum. 33: 847–852.

Lovell, C. R., Burton, J. L. & Horrobin, D. F. (1981) Treatment of atopic eczema with evening primrose oil. Lancet 1: 278.

Morse, P. F., Horrobin, D. F. & Manku, M. S. (1989) Meta-analysis of the placebo-controlled studies of the efficacy of Epogam in the treatment of atopic eczema: relationship between plasma essential fatty acid changes and clinical response. Br. J. Dermatol. 121: 75–90.

Seyberth, H. W., Oelz, O., Kennedy, T., Sweetman, B. J., Danon, A., Frolich, J. C., Heimberg, M. & Oates, J. A. (1975) Increased arachidonate in lipids after administration to man: effects on prostaglandin biosynthesis. Clin. Pharmacol. Ther. 18: 521–529.

Smith, J. B., Ingerman, C., Kocsis, J. J. & Silver, M. J. (1974) Formation of an intermediate in prostaglandin biosynthesis and its association with the platelet release reaction. J. Clin. Investig. 53: 1468–1472.

Tate, G., Mandell, B. F., Laposata, M., Ohliger, D., Baker, D. G., Schumacher, H. R. & Zurier, R. B. (1989) Suppression of acute and chronic inflammation by dietary gamma linolenic acid. J. Rheumatol. 16: 729–733.

Vanderhoek, J. Y., Bryant, R. W. & Bailey, J. M. (1980) Inhibition of leukotriene biosynthesis by the leukocyte product 15-hydroxy-5,8,11,13-eicosatetraenoic acid. J. Biol. Chem. 255: 10064–10066.

Willis, A. L. (1974) An enzymatic mechanism for the antithrombotic and antihemostatic actions of aspirin. Science 183: 325–327.

Ziboh, V. A. & Fletcher, M. P. (1992) Dose-response effects of dietary gammalinolenic acid-enriched oils on human polymorphonuclear-neutrophil biosynthesis of leukotriene B4. Am. J. Clin. Nutr. 55: 39–45.

Zurier, R. B., Rossetti, R. G., Jacobson, E. W., DeMarco, D. M., Liu, N. Y., Temming, J. E., White, B. M. & Laposata, M. (1996) Gamma-linolenic acid treatment of rheumatoid arthritis. A randomized, placebo-controlled trial. Arthritis Rheum. 39: 1808–1817.

References

Introduction

Abeywardena, M.Y., and Head, R.J. 2001. Long chain n-3 polyunsaturated fatty acids and blood vessel function. *Cardiovasc. Res.* **52**:361–371.

American Academy of Allergy, Asthma and Immunology. www.aaaai.org.

American Diabetes Association. www.diabetes.org.

American Heart Association. www.americanheart.org.

Arthritis Foundation. www.arthritis.org.

Asthma and Allergy Foundation of America. www.aafa.org.

Crohn's & Colitis Foundation of America. www.ccfa.org.

Ernst, P., and Suissa, S. 1997. The asthma death problem revisited. *Br. J. Clin. Pharmacol.* **43**:339.

Moore, S., and Simon, J. 1999. The greatest century that ever was. *Policy Analysis* **364**:1–32.

National Center for Chronic Disease Prevention and Health Promotion. www.cdc.gov.

National Institute of Allergy and Infectious Disease. www.niaid.nih.gov.

Rosenstreich, D.L., Eggleston, P., Kattan, M., Baker, D., Slavin, R.G., Gergen, P., Mitchell, H., McNiff-Mortimer, K., Lynn, H., Ownby, D. et al. 1997. The role of cockroach allergy and exposure to cockroach allergen in causing morbidity among inner-city children with asthma. *N. Engl. J. Med.* **336**: 1356–1363.

Ross, R. 1999. Atherosclerosis is an inflammatory disease. *Am. Heart J.* **138**:S419–S420.

Triggiani, M., Granata, F., Giannattasio, G., Borrelli, I., de Paulis, A., and Marone, G. 2003. Lung involvement in rheumatoid arthritis. *Sarcoidosis. Vasc. Diffuse. Lung Dis.* **20(3)**:171–179.

Chapter 1: Diagnosis: Affluenza

Albert, C.M., Campos, H., Stampfer, M.J., Ridker, P.M., Manson, J.E., Willett, W.C., and Ma, J. 2002. Blood levels of long-chain n-3 fatty acids and the risk of sudden death. *N. Engl. J. Med.* **346**:1113–1118.

Asher, M.I., Keil, U., Anderson, H.R., Beasley, R., Crane, J., Martinez, F., Mitchell, E.A., Pearce, N., Sibbald, B., Stewart, A.W. et al. 1995. International Study of Asthma and Allergies in Childhood (ISAAC): rationale and methods. *Eur. Respir. J.* **8**:483–491.

Bach, J.F. 2002. The effect of infections on susceptibility to autoimmune and allergic diseases. *N. Engl. J. Med.* **347**:911–920.

Beasley, R., Pearce, N., and Crane, J. 1997. International trends in asthma mortality. *Ciba Found. Symp.* **206**:140–150.

Beasley, R., Crane, J., Lai, C.K., and Pearce, N. 2000. Prevalence and etiology of asthma. *J. Allergy Clin. Immunol.* **105**:S466–S472.

Beasley, R., Ellwood, P., and Asher, I. 2003. International patterns of the prevalence of pediatric asthma the ISAAC program. *Pediatr. Clin. North Am.* **50**:539–553.

Bjorksten, B., Dumitrascu, D., Foucard, T., Khetsuriani, N., Khaitov, R., Leja, M., Lis, G., Pekkanen, J., Priftanji, A., and Riikjarv, M.A. 1998. Prevalence of childhood asthma, rhinitis and eczema in Scandinavia and Eastern Europe. *Eur. Respir. J.* **12**:432–437.

Bjornsdottir, U.S., and Busse, W.W. 1992. Respiratory infections and asthma. [Review]. *Med. Clin. North Am.* **76**:895–915.

Bodansky, H.J., Staines, A., Stephenson, C., Haigh, D., and Cartwright, R. 1992. Evidence for an environmental effect in the aetiology of insulin dependent diabetes in a transmigratory population. *BMJ* **304**:1020–1022.

Braback, L., Breborowicz, A., Dreborg, S., Knutsson, A., Pieklik, H., and Bjorksten, B. 1994. Atopic sensitization and respiratory symptoms among Polish and Swedish school children. *Clin. Exp. Allergy* **24**:826–835.

Braback, L., Breborowicz, A., Julge, K., Knutsson, A., Riikjarv, M.A., Vasar, M., and Bjorksten, B. 1995. Risk factors for respiratory symptoms and atopic sensitisation in the Baltic area. *Arch. Dis. Child* **72**:487–493.

Burney, P. 1995. The origins of obstructive airways disease. A role for diet? *Am. J. Respir. Crit. Care Med.* **151**:1292–1293.

Burney, P., Malmberg, E., Chinn, S., Jarvis, D., Luczynska, C., and Lai, E. 1997. The distribution of total and specific serum IgE in the European Community Respiratory Health Survey. *J. Allergy Clin. Immunol.* **99**:314–322.

Burr, M.L., Emberlin, J.C., Treu, R., Cheng, S., and Pearce, N.E. 2003. Pollen counts in relation to the prevalence of allergic rhinoconjunctivitis, asthma and atopic eczema in the International Study of Asthma and Allergies in Childhood (ISAAC). *Clin. Exp. Allergy* **33**:1675–1680.

Cookson, J.B. 1987. Prevalence rates of asthma in developing countries and their comparison with those in Europe and North America. *Chest* **91**: 97S–103S.

Dietary supplementation with n-3 polyunsaturated fatty acids and vitamin E after myocardial infarction: results of the GISSI-Prevenzione trial. Gruppo Italiano per lo Studio della Sopravvivenza nell'Infarto miocardico. 1999. *Lancet* **354**:447–455.

Dokholyan, R.S., Albert, C.M., Appel, L.J., Cook, N.R., Whelton, P., and Hennekens, C.H. 2004. A trial of omega-3 fatty acids for prevention of hypertension. *Am. J. Cardiol.* **93**:1041–1043.

Eaton, S.B., Eaton, S.B., III, Konner, M.J., and Shostak, M. 1996. An evolutionary perspective enhances understanding of human nutritional requirements. *J. Nutr.* **126**:1732–1740.

Eaton, S.B., Eaton, S.B., III, and Konner, M.J. 1997. Paleolithic nutrition revisited: a twelve-year retrospective on its nature and implications. *Eur. J. Clin. Nutr.* **51**:207–216.

Eaton, S.B., Eaton, S.B., III, Sinclair, A.J., Cordain, L., and Mann, N.J. 1998. Dietary intake of long-chain polyunsaturated fatty acids during the paleolithic. *World Rev. Nutr. Diet.* **83**:12–23.

Eaton, S.B., and Eaton, S.B., III. 2000. Paleolithic vs. modern diets—selected pathophysiological implications. *Eur. J. Nutr.* **39**:67–70.

Eaton, S.B., Cordain, L., and Eaton, S.B. 2001. An evolutionary foundation for health promotion. *World Rev. Nutr. Diet.* **90**:5–12.

Eaton, S.B., and Eaton, S.B. 2003. An evolutionary perspective on human physical activity: implications for health. *Comp. Biochem. Physiol. A Mol. Integr. Physiol.* **136**:153–159.

El, B.M., Boniface, S., Koscher, V., Mamessier, E., Dupuy, P., Milhe, F., Ramadour, M., Vervloet, D., and Magnan, A. 2003. T cell activation, from atopy to asthma: more a paradox than a paradigm. *Allergy* **58**:844–853.

Ernst, P., and Cormier, Y. 2000. Relative scarcity of asthma and atopy among rural adolescents raised on a farm. *Am. J. Respir. Crit. Care Med.* **161**:1563–1566.

Friedmann, H. 1983. From Peasant to Proletarian—Capitalist development and agrarian transitions—Goodman, D., Redclift, M. *Theory and Society* **12**:539–544.

Friedmann, H. 1985. Health, food, and nutrition in third-world development—Ghosh, Pk. *Contemporary Sociology—A Journal of Reviews* **14**:542–545.

Harris, W.S. 1997. N-3 fatty acids and serum lipoproteins: human studies *Am. J. Clin. Nutr.* **65**:1645S–1654S.

Hotamisligil, G.S. 2000. Molecular mechanisms of insulin resistance and the role of the adipocyte. *Int. J. Obes. Relat. Metab. Disord.* **24 Suppl 4**:S23–S27.

Hotamisligil, G.S. 2003. Inflammatory pathways and insulin action. *Int. J. Obes. Relat. Metab. Disord.* **27 Suppl 3**:S53–S55.

Hu, F.B., Bronner, L., Willett, W.C., Stampfer, M.J., Rexrode, K.M., Albert, C.M., Hunter, D., and Manson, J.E. 2002. Fish and omega-3 fatty acid intake and risk of coronary heart disease in women. *JAMA* **287**:1815–1821.

Hu, F.B., Cho, E., Rexrode, K.M., Albert, C.M., and Manson, J.E. 2003. Fish and long-chain omega-3 fatty acid intake and risk of coronary heart disease and total mortality in diabetic women. *Circulation* **107**:1852–1857.

Jogi, R., Janson, C., Bjornsson, E., Boman, G., and Bjorksten, B. 1996. The prevalence of asthmatic respiratory symptoms among adults in Estonian and Swedish university cities. *Allergy* **51**:331–336.

Jogi, R., Janson, C., Bjornsson, E., Boman, G., and Bjorksten, B. 1998. Atopy and allergic disorders among adults in Tartu, Estonia, compared with Uppsala, Sweden. *Clin. Exp. Allergy* **28**:1072–1080.

Julge, K., Munir, A.K., Vasar, M., and Bjorksten, B. 1998. Indoor allergen levels and other environmental risk factors for sensitization in Estonian homes. *Allergy* **53**:388–393.

Kris-Etherton, P.M., Harris, W.S., and Appel, L.J. 2002. Fish consumption, fish oil, omega-3 fatty acids, and cardiovascular disease. *Circulation* **106**:2747–2757.

Kromann, N., and Green, A. 1980. Epidemiological studies in the Upernavik district, Greenland. Incidence of some chronic diseases 1950–1974. *Acta Med. Scand.* **208**:401–406.

Lewis, S., Hales, S., Slater, T., Pearce, N., Crane, J., and Beasley, R. 1997. Geographical variation in the prevalence of asthma symptoms in New Zealand. *N. Z. Med. J.* **110**:286–289.

Maziak, W. 2002. The hygiene hypothesis and the evolutionary perspective of health. *Prev. Med.* **35**:415–418.

Maziak, W., Behrens, T., Brasky, T.M., Duhme, H., Rzehak, P., Weiland, S.K., and Keil, U. 2003. Are asthma and allergies in children and adolescents increasing? Results from ISAAC phase I and phase III surveys in Munster, Germany. *Allergy* **58**:572–579.

McGeady, S.J. 2004. Immunocompetence and allergy. *Pediatrics* **113**:1107–1113.

Molokhia, M., and McKeigue, P. 2000. Risk for rheumatic disease in relation to ethnicity and admixture. *Arthritis Res.* **2**:115–125.

Molokhia, M., McKeigue, P.M., Cuadrado, M., and Hughes, G. 2001. Systemic lupus erythematosus in migrants from west Africa compared with Afro-Caribbean people in the UK. *Lancet* **357**:1414–1415.

Molokhia, M., Hoggart, C., Patrick, A.L., Shriver, M., Parra, E., Ye, J., Silman, A.J., and McKeigue, P.M. 2003. Relation of risk of systemic lupus erythematosus to west African admixture in a Caribbean population. *Hum. Genet.* **112**:310–318.

Muller, H., de Toledo, F.W., Resch, K.L. Fasting followed by vegetarian diet in patients with rheumatoid arthritis: a systematic review. 2001. *Scand. J. Rheumatol.* **30(1)**:1–10

Murphy, K. 2003. When it comes to fish, go wild. *Business Week,* January 2, 2003.

Nicolai, T., and von Mutius, E. 1996. Respiratory hypersensitivity and environmental factors: East and West Germany. *Toxicol. Lett.* **86**:105–113.

Nicolai, T., and von Mutius, E. 1997. Pollution and the development of allergy: the East and West Germany story. *Arch. Toxicol. Suppl.* **19**:201–206.

Northridge, M.E., Jean-Louis, B., Shoemaker, K., Nicholas, S. 2002. Advancing population health in the Harlem Children's Zone Project. *Soz Praventivmed.* **47(4)**:201–202.

Pearce, N., Sunyer, J., Cheng, S., Chinn, S., Bjorksten, B., Burr, M., Keil, U., Anderson, H.R., and Burney, P. 2000. Comparison of asthma prevalence in the ISAAC and the ECRHS. ISAAC Steering Committee and the European Community Respiratory Health Survey. International Study of Asthma and Allergies in Childhood. *Eur. Respir. J.* **16**:420–426.

Pirotta, Y.F., Mann, N.J., and Kelly, F. 2003. Fatty acid composition of habitual diet. *Asia Pac. J. Clin. Nutr.* **12 Suppl**:S27.

Population Reference Bureau. www.prb.org.

Riikjarv, M.A., Julge, K., Vasar, M., Braback, L., Knutsson, A., and Bjorksten, B. 1995. The prevalence of atopic sensitization and respiratory symptoms among Estonian schoolchildren. *Clin. Exp. Allergy* **25**:1198–1204.

Simon, R.A. 2003. Adverse reactions to food additives. *Curr. Allergy Asthma Rep.* Jan;**3(1)**:62–66.

Strachan, D., Sibbald, B., Weiland, S., it-Khaled, N., Anabwani, G., Anderson, H.R., Asher, M.I., Beasley, R., Bjorksten, B., Burr, M. et al. 1997. Worldwide variations in prevalence of symptoms of allergic rhinoconjunctivitis in children: the International Study of Asthma and Allergies in Childhood (ISAAC). *Pediatr. Allergy Immunol.* **8**:161–176.

U.S. Commodity Rankings. 1998.

Vasar, M., Braback, L., Julge, K., Knutsson, A., Riikjarv, M.A., and Bjorksten, B. 1996. Prevalence of bronchial hyperreactivity as determined by several methods among Estonian schoolchildren. *Pediatr. Allergy Immunol.* **7**:141–146.

von Hertzen, L.C., and Haahtela, T. 2004. Asthma and atopy—the price of affluence? *Allergy* **59**:124–137.

von Mutius, E., Fritzsch, C., Weiland, S.K., Roll, G., and Magnussen, H. 1992.

Prevalence of asthma and allergic disorders among children in united Germany: a descriptive comparison. *BMJ* **305**:1395–1399.

von Mutius, E., Martinez, F.D., Fritzsch, C., Nicolai, T., Roell, G., and Thiemann, H.H. 1994. Prevalence of asthma and atopy in two areas of West and East Germany. *Am. J. Respir. Crit. Care Med.* **149**:358–364.

von Mutius, E. 1996. Epidemiology of asthma: ISAAC—International Study of Asthma and Allergies in Childhood. *Pediatr. Allergy Immunol.* **7**:54–56.

von Mutius, E., Illi, S., Hirsch, T., Leupold, W., Keil, U., and Weiland, S.K. 1999. Frequency of infections and risk of asthma, atopy and airway hyperresponsiveness in children. *Eur. Respir. J.* **14**:4–11.

von Mutius, E. 1999. ISAAC, the world-wide study of asthma and allergies in childhood. *Pneumologie* **53**:101–102.

von Mutius, E. 2001. Infection: friend or foe in the development of atopy and asthma? The epidemiological evidence. *Eur. Respir. J.* **18**:872–881.

von Mutius, E. 2002. Environmental factors influencing the development and progression of pediatric asthma. *J. Allergy Clin. Immunol.* **109**:S525–S532.

von Mutius, E. 2002. Childhood experiences take away your breath as a young adult. *Am. J. Respir. Crit. Care Med.* **165**:1467–1468.

Wahle, K.W., Rotondo, D., and Heys, S.D. 2003. Polyunsaturated fatty acids and gene expression in mammalian systems. *Proc. Nutr. Soc.* **62**:349–360.

Weiss, S.T. 2002. Eat dirt—the hygiene hypothesis and allergic diseases. *N. Engl. J. Med.* **347**:930–931.

Xu, H., Uysal, K.T., Becherer, J.D., Arner, P., and Hotamisligil, G.S. 2002. Altered tumor necrosis factor-alpha (TNF-alpha) processing in adipocytes and increased expression of transmembrane TNF-alpha in obesity. *Diabetes* **51**:1876–1883.

Chapter 2: The War Within

Aiello, R.J., Bourassa, P.A., Lindsey, S., Weng, W., Freeman, A., and Showell, H.J. 2002. Leukotriene B4 receptor antagonism reduces monocytic foam cells in mice. *Arterioscler. Thromb. Vasc. Biol.* **22**:443–449.

Aiello, R.J., Bourassa, P.A., Lindsey, S., Weng, W., Freeman, A., and Showell, H.J. 2002. Leukotriene B4 receptor antagonism reduces monocytic foam cells in mice. *Arterioscler. Thromb. Vasc. Biol.* **22**:443–449.

Bousquet, J., Chanez, P., Lacoste, J.Y., Barneon, G., Ghavanian, N., Enander, I., Venge, P., Ahlstedt, S., Simony-Lafontaine, J., Godard, P. et al. 1990. Eosinophilic inflammation in asthma. *N. Engl. J. Med.* **323**:1033–1039.

Camp, R.D.R., Coutts, A.A., Greaves, M.W., Kay, A.B., and Walport, M.J. 1983. Response of human skin to intradermal injection of leukotrienes C_4, D_4 and B_4. *Br. J. Pharmacol.* **80**:497–502.

Chandran, M., Phillips, S.A., Ciaraldi, T., and Henry, R.R. 2003. Adiponectin: more than just another fat cell hormone? *Diabetes Care* **26**:2442–2450.

Dahlén, S.-E., Hedqvist, P., Hammarström, S., and Samuelsson, B. 1980. Leukotrienes are potent constrictors of human bronchi. *Nature* **288**:484–486.

Drazen, J.M., and Austen, K.F. 1987. Leukotrienes and airway responses. *Am. Rev. Respir. Dis.* **136**:985–998.

Drazen, J.M., O'Brien, J., Sparrow, D., Weiss, S.T., Martins, M.A., Israel, E., and Fanta, C.H. 1992. Recovery of leukotriene E, from the urine of patients with airway obstruction. *Am. Rev. Respir. Dis.* **146**:104–108.

Drazen, J.M. 1998. Leukotrienes as mediators of airway obstruction. *Am. J. Respir. Crit. Care Med.* **158**:S193–S200.

Elmgreen, J., Nielsen, O.H., and Ahnfelt-Ronne, I. 1987. Enhanced capacity for release of leucotriene B_4 by neutrophils in rheumatoid arthritis. *Ann. Rheum. Dis.* **46**:501–505.

Folco, G., Rossoni, G., Buccellati, C., Berti, F., Maclouf, J., and Sala, A. 2000. Leukotrienes in cardiovascular diseases. *Am. J. Respir. Crit. Care Med.* **161**:S112–S116.

Ford-Hutchinson, A.W., Bray, M.A., Doig, M.V., Shipley, M.E., and Smith, M.J.H. 1980. Leukotriene B, a potent chemokinetic and aggregating substance released from polymorphonuclear leukocytes. *Nature* **286**:264–265.

Griffin, M., Weiss, J.W., Leitch, A.G., McFadden, E.R., Jr., Corey, E.J., Austen, K.F., and Drazen, J.M. 1983. Effects of leukotriene D on the airways in asthma. *N. Engl. J. Med.* **308**:436–439.

Hedley, A.A., Ogden, C.L., Johnson, C.L., Carroll, M.D., Curtin, L.R., Flegal, K.M. 2004. Prevalence of overweight and obesity among U.S. children, adolescents, and adults, 1999–2002. *JAMA.* **291(23)**:2847–2850.

Henderson, W.R. 1994. The role of leukotrienes in inflammation. *Ann. Intern. Med.* **121**:684–697.

Holgate, S.T. 1990. Mediator and cellular mechanisms in asthma. *J. R. Coll. Physicians Lond.* **24**:304–317.

Holtzman, M.J. 1991. Arachidonic acid metabolism. Implications of biological chemistry for lung function and disease. *Am. Rev. Respir. Dis.* **143**:188–203.

Lee, T.H., Israel, E., Drazen, J.M., Leitch, A.G., Ravalese, J.I., Corey, E.J., Robinson, D.R., Lewis, R.A., and Austen, K.F. 1986. Enhancement of plasma levels of biologically active leukotriene B compounds during anaphylaxis in guinea pigs pretreated by indomethacin or by a fish oil-enriched diet. *J. Immunol.* **136(7)**:2575–2582.

Samuelsson, B. 1983. Leukotrienes: mediators of hypersensitivity reactions and inflammation. *Science* **220**:568–575.

Smith, C.M., Christie, P.E., Hawksworth, R.J., Thien, F., and Lee, T.H. 1991. Urinary leukotriene E_4 levels following allergen and exercise challenge in bronchial asthma. *Am. Rev. Respir. Dis.* **144**:1411–1413.

Smith, C.M., Hawksworth, R.J., Thien, F.C.K., Christie, P.E., and Lee, T.H. 1992. Urinary leukotriene E_4 in bronchial asthma. *Eur. Respir. J.* **5**:693–699.

Westcott, J.Y., Smith, H.R., Wenzel, S.E., Larsen, G.L., Thomas, R.B., Felsien, D., and Voelkel, N.F. 1991. Urinary leukotriene E_4 in patients with asthma; effect of airways reactivity and sodium cromoglycate. *Am. Rev. Respir. Dis.* **143**:1322–1328.

Chapter 3: The Inflammatory Continuum

Bousquet, J., Chanez, P., Lacoste, J.Y., Barneon, G., Ghavanian, N., Enander, I., Venge, P., Ahlstedt, S., Simony-Lafontaine, J., Godard, P. et al. 1990. Eosinophilic inflammation in asthma. *N. Engl. J. Med.* **323**:1033–1039.

Brown, A.A., and Hu, F.B. 2001. Dietary modulation of endothelial function: implications for cardiovascular disease. *Am. J. Clin. Nutr.* **73**:673–686.

Casserly, I., and Topol, E. 2004. Convergence of atherosclerosis and Alzheimer's disease: inflammation, cholesterol, and misfolded proteins. *Lancet* **363**:1139–1146.

Chandran, M., Phillips, S.A., Ciaraldi, T., and Henry, R.R. 2003. Adiponectin: more than just another fat cell hormone? *Diabetes Care* **26**:2442–2450.

Christie, P.E., Tagari, P., Ford-Hutchinson, A.W., Charlesson, S., Chee, P., Arm, J.P., and Lee, T.H. 1991. Urinary leukotriene E_4 concentrations increase after aspirin challenge in aspirin-sensitive asthmatic subjects. *Am. Rev. Respir. Dis.* **143**:1025–1029.

Cordain, L., Watkins, B.A., and Mann, N.J. 2001. Fatty acid composition and energy density of foods available to African hominids. Evolutionary implications for human brain development. *World Rev. Nutr. Diet.* **90**:144–161.

Coussens, L.M., Werb, Z. 2002. Inflammation and cancer. *Nature.* **420(691)**: 860–867.

Coussens, L.M., Werb, Z. 2001. Inflammatory cells and cancer: think different! *J. Exp. Med.* **193(6)**:F23–26.

Deen, D. 2004. Metabolic syndrome: what is it and what can I do about it? *Am. Fam. Physician* **69**:2887–2888.

Deen, D. 2004. Metabolic syndrome: time for action. *Am. Fam. Physician* **69**:2875–2882.

Diamond, J. 1997. The worst mistake in the history of the human race. *Discovery Magazine.* May:64–66.

Eaton, S.B., Eaton, S.B., III, Konner, M.J., and Shostak, M. 1996. An evolutionary perspective enhances understanding of human nutritional requirements. *J. Nutr.* **126:**1732–1740.

Eaton, S.B., Eaton, S.B., III, and Konner, M.J. 1997. Paleolithic nutrition revisited: a twelve-year retrospective on its nature and implications. *Eur. J. Clin. Nutr.* **51:**207–216.

Eaton, S.B., Eaton, S.B., III, Sinclair, A.J., Cordain, L., and Mann, N.J. 1998. Dietary intake of long-chain polyunsaturated fatty acids during the paleolithic. *World Rev. Nutr. Diet.* **83:**12–23.

Eaton, S.B., and Eaton, S.B., III 2000. Paleolithic vs. modern diets—selected pathophysiological implications. *Eur. J. Nutr.* **39:**67–70.

Eaton, S.B., Cordain, L., and Eaton, S.B. 2001. An evolutionary foundation for health promotion. *World Rev. Nutr. Diet.* **90:**5–12.

Eaton, S.B., and Eaton, S.B. 2003. An evolutionary perspective on human physical activity: implications for health. *Comp. Biochem. Physiol. A Mol. Integr. Physiol.* **136:**153–159.

Global initiative for asthma: global strategy for asthma management and prevention. National Institutes of Health. 2002.

Hotamisligil, G.S. 2000. Molecular mechanisms of insulin resistance and the role of the adipocyte. *Int. J. Obes. Relat. Metab. Disord.* **24 Suppl 4:**S23–S27.

Hotamisligil, G.S. 2003. Inflammatory pathways and insulin action. *Int. J. Obes. Relat. Metab. Disord.* **27 Suppl 3:**S53–S55.

Lemiere, C., Bai, T., Balter, M., Bayliff, C., Becker, A., Boulet, L.P., Bowie, D., Cartier, A., Cave, A., Chapman, K. et al. 2004. Adult asthma consensus guidelines update 2003. *Can. Respir. J.* **11:**9A–18A.

Libby, P., and Simon, D.I. 2001. Inflammation and thrombosis: the clot thickens. *Circulation* **103:**1718–1720.

Libby, P., Ridker, P.M., and Maseri, A. 2002. Inflammation and atherosclerosis. *Circulation* **105:**1135–1143.

Libby, P., and Ridker, P.M. 2004. Inflammation and atherosclerosis: role of C-reactive protein in risk assessment. *Am. J. Med.* **116 Suppl 6A:**S9–S16.

Mann, N.J. 2004. Paleolithic nutrition: what can we learn from the past? *Asia Pac. J. Clin. Nutr.* **13:**S17.

Mehrabian, M., and Allayee, H. 2003. 5-lipoxygenase and atherosclerosis. *Curr. Opin. Lipidol.* **14:**447–457.

Perseghin, G., Petersen, K., and Shulman, G.I. 2003. Cellular mechanism of insulin resistance: potential links with inflammation. *Int. J. Obes. Relat. Metab. Disord.* **27 Suppl 3:**S6–S11.

Schulze, M.B., Rimm, E.B., Shai, I., Rifai, N., and Hu, F.B. 2004. Relationship between adiponectin and glycemic control, blood lipids, and inflammatory markers in men with type 2 diabetes. *Diabetes Care* **27:**1680–1687.

Schulze, M.B., Rimm, E.B., Li, T., Rifai, N., Stampfer, M.J., and Hu, F.B. 2004. C-reactive protein and incident cardiovascular events among men with diabetes. *Diabetes Care* **27**:889–894.

Simopoulos, A.P. 1999. Evolutionary aspects of omega-3 fatty acids in the food supply. *Prostaglandins Leukot. Essent. Fatty Acids* **60**:421–429.

Simopoulos, A.P., and Sidossis, L.S. 2000. What is so special about the traditional diet of Greece: the scientific evidence. *World Rev. Nutr. Diet.* **87**:24–42.

Simopoulos, A.P. 2001. Evolutionary aspects of diet and essential fatty acids. *World Rev. Nutr. Diet.* **88**:18–27.

Simopoulos, A.P. 2001. The Mediterranean diets: what is so special about the diet of Greece? The scientific evidence. *J. Nutr.* **131**:S3065–S3073.

Spanbroek, R., and Habenicht, A.J. 2003. The potential role of antileukotriene drugs in atherosclerosis. *Drug News Perspect.* **16**:485–489.

Sponheimer, M., and Lee-Thorp, J.A. 1999. Isotopic evidence for the diet of an early hominid, Australopithecus africanus. *Science* **283**:368–370.

Steinbaum, S.R. 2004. The metabolic syndrome: an emerging health epidemic in women. *Prog. Cardiovasc. Dis.* **46**:321–336.

Taylor, G.W., Taylor, I., Black, P., Maltby, N.H., Turner, N., Fuller, R.W., and Dollery, C.T. 1989. Urinary leukotriene E_4 after antigen challenge and in acute asthma and allergic rhinitis. *Lancet* **1**:584–588.

Weiss, S.T., and Shore, S. 2004. Obesity and asthma: directions for research. *Am. J. Respir. Crit. Care Med.* **169**:963–968.

Wellen, K.E., and Hotamisligil, G.S. 2003. Obesity-induced inflammatory changes in adipose tissue. *J. Clin. Invest.* **112**:1785–1788.

Wenzel, S.E. 2000. *Asthma and the small airways.* S.P. Peters, editor. American Thoracic Society, New York.

Xu, H., Uysal, K.T., Becherer, J.D., Arner, P., and Hotamisligil, G.S. 2002. Altered tumor necrosis factor-alpha (TNF-alpha) processing in adipocytes and increased expression of transmembrane TNF-alpha in obesity. *Diabetes* **51**:1876–1883.

Yeh, E.T. 2004. C-reactive protein is an essential aspect of cardiovascular risk factor stratification. *Can. J. Cardiol.* **20**:93B–96B.

Yeh, E.T. 2004. CRP as a mediator of disease. *Circulation* **109**:II11–II14.

Chapter 4: The Billion-Dollar Pathway

Borgeat, P., and Samuelsson, B. 1979. Metabolism of arachidonic acid by polymorphonuclear leukocytes: structural analysis of novel hydroxylated compounds. *J. Biol. Chem.* **254**:7865–7869.

Borgeat, P., and Samuelsson, B. 1979. Arachidonic acid metabolism in polymorphonuclear leukocytes: unstable intermediate in the formation of dihydroxy acids. *Proc. Natl. Acad. Sci. U.S.A.* **76**:3213–3217.

Borgeat, P., and Samuelsson, B. 1979. Transformation of arachidonic acid by rabbit polymorphonuclear leukocytes: formation of a novel dihydroxyeicosatetraenoic acid. *J. Biol. Chem.* **254**:2643–2646.

Chilton, F.H., Connell, T.R. 1988. 1-ether-linked phosphoglycerides: major endogenous sources of arachidonate in the human neutrophil. *J. Biol. Chem.* Apr **15;263(11)**:5260–5265.

Chilton, F.H. 1989. Potential phospholipid source(s) of arachidonate used for the synthesis of leukotrienes by the human neutrophil. *Biochem. J.* Mar **1;258(2)**: 327–333.

Chilton, F.H., Murphy, R.C. 1986. Remodeling of arachidonate-containing phosphoglycerides within the human neutrophil. *J. Biol. Chem.* **261(17)**: 7771–7777.

Hui, K.P., Taylor, I.K., Taylor, G.W., Rubin, P., Kesterson, J., Barnes, N.C., and Barnes, P.J. 1991. Effect of a 5-lipoxygenase inhibitor on leukotriene generation and airway responses after allergen challenge in asthmatic patients. *Thorax* **46**:184–189.

Lane, S.J., Palmer, J.B.D., Skidmore, I.F., and Lee, T.H. 1990. Corticosteroid pharmacokinetics in asthma. *Lancet* **336**:1265.

Larsen, J.S., and Acosta, E.P. 1993. Leukotriene-receptor antagonists and 5-lipoxygenase inhibitors in asthma. *Ann. Pharmacother.* **27**:898–903.

Murphy, R.C., Hammarstrom, S., and Samuelsson, B. 1979. Leukotriene C: a slow-reacting substance from murine mastocytoma cells. *Proc. Natl. Acad. Sci. U.S.A.* **76(9)**:4275–4279.

O'Banion, M.K., Winn, V.D., Young, D.A. 1992. cDNA cloning and functional activity of a glucocorticoid-regulated inflammatory cyclooxygenase. *Proc. Natl. Acad. Sci. USA.* **89(11)**:4888–4892.

O'Sullivan, M.G., Chilton, F.H., Huggins, E.M., Jr., McCall, C.E. 1992. Lipopolysaccharide priming of alveolar macrophages for enhanced synthesis of prostanoids involves induction of a novel prostaglandin H synthase. *J. Biol Chem.* **267(21)**:14547–14550.

Rouzer, C.A., Matsumoto, T., and Samuelsson, B. 1986. Single protein from human leukocytes possesses 5-lipoxygenase and leukotriene A_4 synthase activities. *Proc. Natl. Acad. Sci. U.S.A.* **83**:857–861.

Samuelsson, B., Borgeat, P., Hammarstrom, S., Murphy, R.C. 1980. Leukotrienes: a new group of biologically active compounds. *Adv. Prostaglandin Thromboxane Leukot. Res.* **6**:1–18.

Schleimer, R.P. 1993. Glucocorticosteroids. In *Allergy, Principles and Practice.*

E. Middleton, Jr., Reed, C.E., Ellis, E.F., Adkinson, N.F., Jr., Yunginger, J.W., and Busse, W.W., editors. Mosby. St Louis. 893–925.

Surette, M.E., Koumenis, I.L., Edens, M.B., Tramposch, K.M., Clayton, B., Bowton, D., and Chilton, F.H. 2003. Inhibition of leukotriene biosynthesis by a novel dietary fatty acid formulation in patients with atopic asthma: a randomized, placebo-controlled, parallel-group, prospective trial. *Clin. Ther.* **25:**972–979.

Vane, J. 1994. Towards a better aspirin. *Nature* **367:**215–216.

Vane, J.R., and Botting, R.M. 1998. Anti-inflammatory drugs and their mechanism of action. *Inflamm. Res.* **47:**S78–S87.

Venkatesh, V.C., and Ballard, P.L. 1991. Glucocorticoids and gene expression. *Am. J. Respir. Cell Mol. Biol.* **4:**301–303.

Chapter 5: Closing in on the Culprit

Burdge, G.C., Jones, A.E., and Wootton, S.A. 2002. Eicosapentaenoic and docosapentaenoic acids are the principal products of alpha-linolenic acid metabolism in young men. *Br. J. Nutr.* **88:**355–363.

Burdge, G.C., Finnegan, Y.E., Minihane, A.M., Williams, C.M., and Wootton, S.A. 2003. Effect of altered dietary n-3 fatty acid intake upon plasma lipid fatty acid composition, conversion of [13C]alpha-linolenic acid to longer-chain fatty acids and partitioning towards beta-oxidation in older men. *Br. J. Nutr.* **90:**311–321.

Cho, H.P., Nakamura, M., and Clarke, S.D. 1999. Cloning, expression, and fatty acid regulation of the human delta-5 desaturase. *J. Biol. Chem.* **274:** 37335–37339.

Cho, H.P., Nakamura, M.T., and Clarke, S.D. 1999. Cloning, expression, and nutritional regulation of the mammalian delta-6 desaturase. *J. Biol. Chem.* **274:**471–477.

Dwyer, J.H., Wu, H.Y., Dwyer, K.M., Allayee, H., Lusis, A.J., and Mehrabian, M. 2003. Dietary arachidonic acid and linoleic acid are atherogenic while fish oils are protective, in a variant 5-lipoxygenase promoter genotype. *Circulation* **107:**E7003.

Dwyer, J.H., Allayee, H., Dwyer, K.M., Fan, J., Wu, H.Y., Mar, R., Lusis, A.J., and Mehrabian, M. 2004. Arachidonate 5-lipoxygenase promoter genotype, dietary arachidonic acid, and atherosclerosis. *N. Engl. J. Med.* **350:**29–37.

Ferretti, A., Nelson, G.J., Schmidt, P.C., Kelley, D.S., Bartolini, G., and Flanagan, V.P. 1997. Increased dietary arachidonic acid enhances the synthesis of vasoactive eicosanoids in humans. *Lipids* **32:**435–439.

Helgadottir, A., Manolescu, A., Thorleifsson, G., Gretarsdottir, S., Jonsdottir,

H., Thorsteinsdottir, U., Samani, N.J., Gudmundsson, G., Grant, S.F.A., Thorgeirsson, G. et al. 2004. The gene encoding 5-lipoxygenase activating protein confers risk of myocardial infarction and stroke. *Nat. Genet.* **36:** 233–239.

High, K.P., Sinclair, J., Easter, L.H., Case, D., Chilton, F.H. 2003. Advanced age, but not anergy, is associated with altered serum polyunsaturated fatty acid levels. *J. Nutr. Health Aging* **7(6):**378–384.

Innis, S.M., and Elias, S.L. 2003. Intakes of essential n-6 and n-3 polyunsaturated fatty acids among pregnant Canadian women. *Am. J. Clin. Nutr.* **77:** 473–478.

Jump, D.B. 2002. The biochemistry of n-3 polyunsaturated fatty acids. *J. Biol. Chem.* **277:**8755–8758.

Kelley, D.S., Nelson, G.J., Love, J.E., Branch, L.B., Taylor, P.C., Schmidt, P.C., Mackey, B.E., and Iacono, J.M. 1993. Dietary alpha-linolenic acid alters tissue fatty acid composition, but not blood lipids, lipoproteins or coagulation status in humans. *Lipids* **28:**533–537.

Kelley, D.S., Taylor, P.C., Nelson, G.J., Schmidt, P.C., Mackey, B.E., and Kyle, D. 1997. Effects of dietary arachidonic acid on human immune response. *Lipids* **32:**449–456.

Kelley, D.S. 2001. Modulation of human immune and inflammatory responses by dietary fatty acids. *Nutrition* **17:**669–673.

Li, D., Ng, A., Mann, N.J., and Sinclair, A.J. 1998. Contribution of meat fat to dietary arachidonic acid. *Lipids* **33:**437–440.

Mehrabian, M., Allayee, H., Wong, J., Shi, W., Wang, X.P., Shaposhnik, Z., Funk, C.D., Lusis, A.J., and Shih, W. 2002. Identification of 5-lipoxygenase as a major gene contributing to atherosclerosis susceptibility in mice. *Circ. Res.* **91:**120–126.

Mehrabian, M., and Allayee, H. 2003. 5-Lipoxygenase and atherosclerosis. *Curr. Opin. Lipidol.* **14:**447–457.

Meyer, B.J., Mann, N.J., Lewis, J.L., Milligan, G.C., Sinclair, A.J., and Howe, P.R. 2003. Dietary intakes and food sources of omega-6 and omega-3 polyunsaturated fatty acids *Lipids* **38:**391–398.

Murray, M.J., Kumar, M., Gregory, T.J., Banks, P.L., Tazelaar, H.D., and DeMichele, S.J. 1995. Select dietary fatty acids attenuate cardiopulmonary dysfunction during acute lung injury in pigs. *Am. J. Physiol.* **269:**H2090–H2099.

Parker-Barnes, J.M., Das, T., Bobik, E., Leonard, A.E., Thurmond, J.M., Chaung, L.T., Huang, Y.S., and Mukerji, P. 2000. Identification and characterization of an enzyme involved in the elongation of n-6 and n-3 polyunsaturated fatty acids. *Proc. Natl. Acad. Sci. U.S.A.* **97:**8284–8289.

Pawlosky, R.J., Hibbeln, J.R., Novotny, J.A., and Salem, N., Jr. 2001. Physiological compartmental analysis of alpha-linolenic acid metabolism in adult humans. *J. Lipid Res.* **42**:1257–1265.

Pischon, T., Hankinson, S.E., Hotamisligil, G.S., Rifai, N., Willett, W.C., and Rimm, E.B. 2003. Habitual dietary intake of n-3 and n-6 fatty acids in relation to inflammatory markers among U.S. men and women. *Circulation* **108**:155–160.

Salem, N., Jr., and Pawlosky, R.J. 1994. Arachidonate and docosahexaenoate biosynthesis in various species and compartments in vivo. *World Rev. Nutr. Diet.* **75**:114–119.

Salem, N., Jr., Pawlosky, R., Wegher, B., and Hibbeln, J. 1999. In vivo conversion of linoleic acid to arachidonic acid in human adults. *Prostaglandins Leukot. Essent. Fatty Acids* **60**:407–410.

Seyberth, H.W., Oelz, O., Kennedy, T., Sweetman, B.J., Danon, A., Frolich, J.C., Heimberg, M., and Oates, J.A. 1975. Increased arachidonate in lipids after administration to man: effects on prostaglandin biosynthesis. *Clin. Pharmacol. Ther.* **18**:521–529.

Sinclair, A.J., and Mann, N.J. 1996. Short-term diets rich in arachidonic acid influence plasma phospholipid polyunsaturated fatty acid levels and prostacyclin and thromboxane production in humans. *J. Nutr.* **126**:S1110–S1114.

Singer, P., Berger, I., Wirth, M., Godicke, W., Jaeger, W., and Voigt, S. 1986. Slow desaturation and elongation of linoleic and alpha-linolenic acids as a rationale of eicosapentaenoic acid-rich diet to lower blood pressure and serum lipids in normal, hypertensive and hyperlipemic subjects. *Prostaglandins Leukot. Med.* **24**:173–193.

Spanbroek, R., Grabner, R., Lotzer, K., Hildner, M., Urbach, A., Ruhling, K., Moos, M.P., Kaiser, B., Cohnert, T.U., Wahlers, T. et al. 2003. Expanding expression of the 5-lipoxygenase pathway within the arterial wall during human atherogenesis. *Proc. Natl. Acad. Sci. U.S.A.* **100**:1238–1243.

Ticono, J. 1982. Dietary requirements and functions of alpha-linolenic acid in animals. *Prog. Lipid. Res.* **21**:1–45.

Whelan, J., Surette, M.E., Hardardottir, I., Lu, G., Golemboski, K.A., Larsen, E., and Kinsella, J.E. 1993. Dietary arachidonate enhances tissue arachidonate levels and eicosanoid production in Syrian hamsters. *J. Nutr.* **123**:2174–2185.

Yamazaki, K., Fujikawa, M., Hamazaki, T., Yano, S., and Shono, T. 1992. Comparison of the conversion rates of alpha-linolenic acid (18:3[n-3]) and stearidonic acid (18:4[n-3]) to longer polyunsaturated fatty acids in rats. *Biochim. Biophys. Acta* **1123**:18–26.

Yu, G., and Bjorksten, B. 1998. Polyunsaturated fatty acids in school children in relation to allergy and serum IgE levels. *Pediatr. Allergy Immunol.* **9**:133–138.

Chapter 6: Toxic Superfoods

Allman, M.A., Pena, M.M., and Pang, D. 1995. Supplementation with flaxseed oil versus sunflower seed oil in healthy young men consuming a low fat diet: effects on platelet composition and function. *Eur. J. Clin. Nutr* **49**:169–178.

Burdge, G.C., Jones, A.E., and Wootton, S.A. 2002. Eicosapentaenoic and docosapentaenoic acids are the principal products of alpha-linolenic acid metabolism in young men. *Br. J. Nutr.* **88**:355–363.

Burdge, G.C., Finnegan, Y.E., Minihane, A.M., Williams, C.M., and Wootton, S.A. 2003. Effect of altered dietary n-3 fatty acid intake upon plasma lipid fatty acid composition, conversion of (13C)alpha-linolenic acid to longer-chain fatty acids and partitioning towards beta-oxidation in older men. *Br. J. Nutr.* **90**:311–321.

Cho, H.P., Nakamura, M., and Clarke, S.D. 1999. Cloning, expression, and nutritional regulation of the human delta-5 desaturase. *J. Biol. Chem.* **274**:37335–37339.

Cho, H.P., Nakamura, M.T., and Clarke, S.D. 1999. Cloning, expression, and nutritional regulation of the mammalian delta-6 desaturase. *J. Biol. Chem.* **274**:471–477.

Clay, C.E., Atsumi, G.I., High, K.P., and Chilton, F.H. 2001. Early *de novo* gene expression is required for 15-Deoxy-Delta [12,14] prostaglandin J$_2$-induced apoptosis in breast cancer cells. *J. Biol. Chem.* **276**:47131–47135.

Duchen, K., Yu, G., and Bjorksten, B. 1998. Atopic sensitization during the first year of life in relation to long chain polyunsaturated fatty acid levels in human milk. *Pediatr. Res.* **44**:478–484.

Dwyer, J.H., Wu, H.Y., Dwyer, K.M., Allayee, H., Lusis, A.J., and Mehrabian, M. 2003. Dietary arachidonic acid and linoleic acid are atherogenic while fish oils are protective, in a variant 5-lipoxygenase promoter genotype. *Circulation* **107**:E7003.

Dwyer, J.H., Allayee, H., Dwyer, K.M., Fan, J., Wu, H.Y., Mar, R., Lusis, A.J., and Mehrabian, M. 2004. Arachidonate 5-lipoxygenase promoter genotype, dietary arachidonic acid, and atherosclerosis. *N. Engl. J. Med.* **350**:29–37.

Ferretti, A., Nelson, G.J., Schmidt, P.C., Kelley, D.S., Bartolini, G., and Flanagan, V.P. 1997. Increased dietary arachidonic acid enhances the synthesis of vasoactive eicosanoids in humans. *Lipids* **32**:435–439.

Guichardant, M., Traitler, H., Spielmann, D., Sprecher, H., and Finot, P.A. 1993. Stearidonic acid, an inhibitor of the 5-lipoxygenase pathway: a comparison with timnodonic and dihomogammalinolenic acid. *Lipids* **28**:321–324.

Helgadottir, A., Manolescu, A., Thorleifsson, G., Gretarsdottir, S., Jonsdottir, H., Thorsteinsdottir, U., Samani, N.J., Gudmundsson, G., Grant, S.F.A., Thorgeirsson, G. et al. 2004. The gene encoding 5-lipoxygenase activating protein confers risk of myocardial infarction and stroke. *Nat. Genet.* **36**:233–239.

Innis, S.M., and Elias, S.L. 2003. Intakes of essential n-6 and n-3 polyunsaturated fatty acids among pregnant Canadian women. *Am. J. Clin. Nutr.* **77**:473–478.

Ishihara, K., Komatsu, W., Saito, H., and Shinohara, K. 2002. Comparison of the effects of dietary alpha-linolenic, stearidonic, and eicosapentaenoic acids on production of inflammatory mediators in mice. *Lipids* **37**:481–486.

James, M.J., Ursin, V.M., and Cleland, L.G. 2003. Metabolism of stearidonic acid in human subjects: comparison with the metabolism of other n-3 fatty acids. *Am. J. Clin. Nutr.* **77**:1140–1145.

Jump, D.B. 2002. The biochemistry of n-3 polyunsaturated fatty acids. *J. Biol. Chem.* **277**:8755–8758.

Kelley, D.S., Nelson, G.J., Love, J.E., Branch, L.B., Taylor, P.C., Schmidt, P.C., Mackey, B.E., and Iacono, J.M. 1993. Dietary alpha-linolenic acid alters tissue fatty acid composition, but not blood lipids, lipoproteins or coagulation status in humans. *Lipids* **28**:533–537.

Kelley, D.S., Taylor, P.C., Nelson, G.J., Schmidt, P.C., Mackey, B.E., and Kyle, D. 1997. Effects of dietary arachidonic acid on human immune response. *Lipids* **32**:449–456.

Kelley, D.S. 2001. Modulation of human immune and inflammatory responses by dietary fatty acids. *Nutrition* **17**:669–673.

Layne, K.S., Goh, Y.K., Jumpsen, J.A., Ryan, E.A., Chow, P., and Clandinin, M.T. 1996. Normal subjects consuming physiological levels of 18:3(n-3) and 20:5(n-3) from flaxseed or fish oils have characteristic differences in plasma lipid and lipoprotein fatty acid levels. *J. Nutr.* **126**:2130–2140.

Li, D., Ng, A., Mann, N.J., and Sinclair, A.J. 1998. Contribution of meat fat to dietary arachidonic acid. *Lipids* **33**:437–440.

Mantzioris, E., James, M.J., Gibson, R.A., and Cleland, L.G. 1994. Dietary substitution with an alpha-linolenic acid-rich vegetable oil increases eicosapentaenoic acid concentrations in tissues. *Am. J. Clin. Nutr.* **59**:1304–1309.

Mehrabian, M., Allayee, H., Wong, J., Shi, W., Wang, X.P., Shaposhnik, Z., Funk, C.D., Lusis, A.J., and Shih, W. 2002. Identification of 5-lipoxygenase as a major gene contributing to atherosclerosis susceptibility in mice. *Circ. Res.* **91**:120–126.

Parker-Barnes, J.M., Das, T., Bobik, E., Leonard, A.E., Thurmond, J.M., Chaung, L.T., Huang, Y.S., and Mukerji, P. 2000. Identification and characterization of an enzyme involved in the elongation of n-6 and n-3 polyunsaturated fatty acids. *Proc. Natl. Acad. Sci. U.S.A.* **97**:8284–8289.

Pawlosky, R.J., Hibbeln, J.R., Novotny, J.A., and Salem, N., Jr. 2001. Physiological compartmental analysis of alpha-linolenic acid metabolism in adult humans. *J. Lipid Res.* **42**:1257–1265.

Pawlosky, R.J., Hibbeln, J.R., Lin, Y., Goodson, S., Riggs, P., Sebring, N., Brown, G.L., and Salem, N., Jr. 2003. Effects of beef- and fish-based diets on the kinetics of n-3 fatty acid metabolism in human subjects. *Am. J. Clin. Nutr.* **77**:565–572.

Petrik, M.B., McEntee, M.F., Johnson, B.T., Obukowicz, M.G., and Whelan, J. 2000. Highly unsaturated (n-3) fatty acids, but not alpha-linolenic, conjugated linoleic or gamma-linolenic acids, reduce tumorigenesis in Apc (Min/+) mice. *J. Nutr.* **130**:2434–2443.

Salem, N., Jr., and Pawlowsky, R.J. 1994. Arachidonate and docosahexaenoate biosynthesis in various species and compartments in vivo. *World Rev. Nutr. Diet.* **75**:114–119.

Salem, N., Jr., Pawlosky, R., Wegher, B., and Hibbeln, J. 1999. In vivo conversion of linoleic acid to arachidonic acid in human adults. *Prostaglandins Leukot. Essent. Fatty Acids* **60**:407–410.

Seyberth, H.W., Oelz, O., Kennedy, T., Sweetman, B.J., Danon, A., Frolich, J.C., Heimberg, M., and Oates, J.A. 1975. Increased arachidonate in lipids after administration to man: effects on prostaglandin biosynthesis. *Clin. Pharmacol. Ther.* **18**:521–529.

Sinclair, A.J., and Mann, N.J. 1996. Short-term diets rich in arachidonic acid influence plasma phospholipid polyunsaturated fatty acid levels and prostacyclin and thromboxane production in humans. *J. Nutr.* **126**:S1110–S1114.

Singer, P., Berger, I., Wirth, M., Godicke, W., Jaeger, W., and Voigt, S. 1986. Slow desaturation and elongation of linoleic and alpha-linolenic acids as a rationale of eicosapentaenoic acid-rich diet to lower blood pressure and serum lipids in normal, hypertensive and hyperlipemic subjects. *Prostaglandis Leukot. Med.* **24**:173–193.

Surette, M.E., Edens, M., Chilton, F.H., and Tramposch, K.M. 2004. Dietary echium oil increases plasma and neutrophil long-chain (n-3) fatty acids and lowers serum triacylglycerols in hypertriglyceridemic humans. *J. Nutr.* **134**:1406–1411.

Uauy, R., Hoffman, D.R., Mena, P., Llanos, A., and Birch, E.E. 2003. Term infant studies of DHA and ARA supplementation on neurodevelopment: results of randomized controlled trials. *J. Pediatr.* **143**:S17–S25.

Uauy, R., and Castillo, C. 2003. Lipid requirements of infants: implications for nutrient composition of fortified complementary foods. *J. Nutr.* **133**: 2962S–2972S.

Ursin, V.M. 2003. Modification of plant lipids for human health: development of functional land-based omega-3 fatty acids. *J. Nutr.* **133**:4271–4274.

Wensing, A.G., Mensink, R.P., and Hornstra, G. 1999. Effects of dietary n-3 polyunsaturated fatty acids from plant and marine origin on platelet aggregation in healthy elderly subjects. *Br. J. Nutr.* **82**:183–191.

Yamazaki, K., Fujikawa, M., Hamazaki, T., Yano, S., and Shono, T. 1992. Comparison of the conversion rates of alpha-linolenic acid (18:3[n-3]) and stearidonic acid (18:4[n-3]) to longer polyunsaturated fatty acids in rats. *Biochim. Biophys. Acta* **1123**:18–26.

Yu, G., Duchen, K., and Bjorksten, B. 1998. Fatty acid composition in colostrum and mature milk from non-atopic and atopic mothers during the first 6 months of lactation. *Acta Paediatr.* **87**:729–736.

Yu, G., and Bjorksten, B. 1998. Serum levels of phospholipid fatty acids in mothers and their babies in relation to allergic disease. *Eur. J. Pediatr.* **157**: 298–303.

Yu, G., and Bjorksten, B. 1998. Polyunsaturated fatty acids in school children in relation to allergy and serum IgE levels. *Pediatr. Allergy Immunol.* **9**:133–138.

Chapter 7: Bringing Overactive Inflammation Back into Balance

Arm, J.P., Horton, C.E., Mencia-Huerta, J.-M., House, F., Eiser, N.M., Clark, T.J.H., Spur, B.W., and Lee, T.H. 1988. Effect of dietary supplementation with fish oil lipids on mild asthma. *Thorax* **43**:84–92.

Arm, J.P., Horton, C.E., Spur, B.W., Mencia-Huerta, J.-M., and Lee, T.H. 1989. The effects of dietary supplementation with fish oil lipids on the airways response to inhaled allergen in bronchial asthma. *Am. Rev. Respir. Dis.* **139**:1395–1400.

Barham, J.B., Edens, M.B., Fonteh, A.N., Johnson, M.M., Easter, L., and Chilton, F.H. 2000. Addition of eicosapentaenoic acid to gamma-linolenic acid-supplemented diets prevents serum arachidonic acid accumulation in humans. *J. Nutr.* **130**:1925–1931.

Chapkin, R.S., Somers, S.D., and Erickson, K.L. 1988. Dietary manipulation of macrophage phospholipid classes: selective increase of dihomogamma-linolenic acid. *Lipids* **23**:766–770.

Chapkin, R.S., Miller, C.C., Somers, S.D., and Erickson, K.L. 1988. Ability of 15-hydroxyeicosatrienoic acid (15-OH-20:3) to modulate macrophage arachidonic acid metabolism. *Biochem. Biophys. Res. Commun.* **153**:799–804.

Chapkin, R.S., and Coble, K.J. 1991. Utilization of gammalinolenic acid by mouse peritoneal macrophages. *Biochim. Biophys. Acta* **1085**:365–370.

Chilton, F.H., Patel, M., Fonteh, A.N., Hubbard, W.C., and Triggiani, M. 1993. Dietary n-3 fatty-acid effects on neutrophil lipid-composition and mediator production-influence of duration and dosage. *J. Clin. Invest.* **91**: 115–122.

Chilton, L., Surette, M.E., Swan, D.D., Fonteh, A.N., Johnson, M.M., and Chilton, F.H. 1996. Metabolism of gammalinolenic acid in human neutrophils. *J. Immunol.* **156**:2941–2947.

Christophe, A., Robberecht, E., Franckx, H., De Baets, F., and van de Pas, M. 1994. Effect of administration of gamma-linolenic acid on the fatty acid composition of serum phospholipids and cholesteryl esters in patients with cystic fibrosis. *Ann. Nutr. Metab.* **38**:40–47.

Dooper, M.M., van Riel, B., Graus, Y.M., and M'Rabet, L. 2003. Dihomo-gamma-linolenic acid inhibits tumour necrosis factor-alpha production by human leucocytes independently of cyclooxygenase activity. *Immunology* **110**:348–357.

Eaton, S.B., Eaton, S.B., III, Konner, M.J., and Shostak, M. 1996. An evolutionary perspective enhances understanding of human nutritional requirements. *J. Nutr.* **126**:1732–1740.

Eaton, S.B., Eaton, S.B., III, and Konner, M.J. 1997. Paleolithic nutrition revisited: a twelve-year retrospective on its nature and implications. *Eur. J. Clin. Nutr.* **51**:207–216.

Eaton, S.B., Eaton, S.B., III, Sinclair, A.J., Cordain, L., and Mann, N.J. 1998. Dietary intake of long-chain polyunsaturated fatty acids during the paleolithic. *World Rev. Nutr. Diet.* **83**:12–23.

Eaton, S.B., and Eaton, S.B., III. 2000. Paleolithic vs. modern diets—selected pathophysiological implications. *Eur. J. Nutr.* **39**:67–70.

Eaton, S.B., Cordain, L., and Eaton, S.B. 2001. An evolutionary foundation for health promotion. *World Rev. Nutr. Diet.* **90**:5–12.

Eaton, S.B., and Eaton, S.B. 2003. An evolutionary perspective on human physical activity: implications for health. *Comp Biochem. Physiol. A Mol. Integr. Physiol.* **136**:153–159.

Fan, Y.Y., Ramos, K.S., and Chapkin, R.S. 1997. Dietary gamma-linolenic acid enhances mouse macrophage-derived prostaglandin E1 which inhibits vascular smooth muscle cell proliferation. *J. Nutr.* **127**:1765–1771.

Fan, Y.Y., Ramos, K.S., and Chapkin, R.S. 1999. Modulation of atherogenesis by dietary gamma-linolenic acid. *Adv. Exp. Med. Biol.* **469**:485–491.

Fletcher, M.P., and Ziboh, V.A. 1990. Effects of dietary supplementation with eicosapentaenoic acid or gamma-linolenic acid on neutrophil phospholipid fatty acid composition and activation responses. *Inflammation* **14**:585–597.

Forman, B.M., Tontonoz, P., Chen, J., Brun, R.P., Spiegelman, B.M., and Evans, R.M. 1995. 15-Deoxy-delta 12, 14-prostaglandin J_2 is a ligand for the adipocyte determination factor PPAR gamma. *Cell* **83**:803–812.

Goldman, D.W., Pickett, W.C., and Goetzl, E.J. 1983. Human neutrophil chemotactic and degranulating activities of leukotriene B_5 (LTB_5) derived from eicosapentaenoic acid. *Biochem. Biophys. Res. Commun.* **117**:282–288.

Guil-Guerrero, J.L., Gomez-Mercado, F., Garcia-Maroto, F., and Campra-Madrid, P. 2000. Occurrence and characterization of oils rich in gamma-linolenic acid Part I: echium seeds from Macaronesia. *Phytochemistry* **53**:451–456.

Harbige, L.S., Layward, L., Morris-Downes, M.M., Dumonde, D.C., and Amor, S. 2000. The protective effects of omega-6 fatty acids in experimental autoimmune encephalomyelitis (EAE) in relation to transforming growth factor-beta 1 (TGF-beta1) up-regulation and increased prostaglandin E2 (PGE2) production. *Clin. Exp. Immunol.* **122**:445–452.

Hirafuji, M., Machida, T., Tsunoda, M., Miyamoto, A., and Minami, M. 2002. Docosahexaenoic acid potentiates interleukin-1b induction of nitric oxide synthase through mechanism involving p44/42 MAPK activation in rat vascular smooth muscle cells. *Br. J. Pharmacol.* **136**:613–619.

Johnson, M.M., Swan, D.D., Surette, M.E., Stegner, J., Chilton, T., Fonteh, A.N., and Chilton, F.H. 1997. Dietary supplementation with gamma-linolenic acid alters fatty acid content and eicosanoid production in healthy humans. *J. Nutr.* **127**:1435–1444.

Layne, K.S., Goh, Y.K., Jumpsen, J.A., Ryan, E.A., Chow, P., and Clandinin, M.T. 1996. Normal subjects consuming physiological levels of 18:3(n-3) and 20:5(n-3) from flaxseed or fish oils have characteristic differences in plasma lipid and lipoprotein fatty acid levels. *J. Nutr.* **126**:2130–2140.

Lee, T.H., Mencia-Huerta, J.M., Shih, C., Corey, E.J., Lewis, R.A., and Austen, K.F. 1984. Characterization and biological properties of 5,12-dihydroxy derivatives of eicosapentaenoic acid including leukotriene B_5 and the double lipoxygenase product. *J. Biol. Chem.* **259**:2383–2389.

Lee, T.H., Mencia-Huerta, J.M., Shih, C., Corey, E.J., Lewis, R.A., and Austen, K.F. 1984. Effects of exogenous arachidonic, eicosapentaenoic, and docosahexaenoic acids on the generation of 5-lipoxygenase pathway products by ionophore-activated human neutrophils. *J. Clin. Invest.* **74**:1922–1933.

Lee, T.H., Hoover, R.L., Williams, J.D., Sperling, R.I., Ravelese, J., Spur, B.W., Robinson, D.R., Corey, E.J., Lewis, R.A., and Austen, K.F. 1985. Effect of dietary enrichment with eicosapentaenoic and docosahexaenoic acid on *in vitro* neutrophil and monocyte leukotriene generation and neutrophil function. *N. Engl. J. Med.* **312**:1217–1224.

Lee, T.H., Austen,K.F., Leitch, A.G., Israel, E., Robinson, D.R., Lewis, R.A., Corey, E.J., and Drazen, J.M. 1985. The effects of a fish-oil enriched diet on pulmonary mechanics during anaphylaxis. *Am. Rev. Respir. Dis.* **132**:1204–1209.

Lee, T.H., and Arm, J.P. 1986. Prospects for modifying the allergic response by fish oil diets. *Clin. Allergy* **16**:89–100.

Leventhal, L.J., Boyce, E.G., and Zurier, R.B. 1993. Treatment of rheumatoid arthritis with gammalinolenic acid. *Ann. Intern. Med.* **119**:867–873.

Lopez-Garcia, E., Schulze, M.B., Manson, J.E., Meigs, J.B., Albert, C.M., Rifai, N., Willett, W.C., and Hu, F.B. 2004. Consumption of (n-3) fatty acids is related to plasma biomarkers of inflammation and endothelial activation in women. *J. Nutr.* **134**:1806–1811.

Pek, S.B., Nathan, M.H. 1994. Role of eicosanoids in biosynthesis and secretion of inslin. *Diabete. Metab.* **20(2)**:146–149.

Petrik, M.B., McEntee, M.F., Johnson, B.T., Obukowicz, M.G., and Whelan, J. 2000. Highly unsaturated (n-3) fatty acids, but not alpha-linolenic, conjugated linoleic or gamma-linolenic acids, reduce tumorigenesis in Apc (Min/+) mice. *J. Nutr.* **130**:2434–2443.

Picado, C., Castillo, J.A., Schinca, N., Pujades, M., Ordinas, A., Coronas, A., and Agusti-Vidal, A. 1988. Effects of a fish oil enriched diet on aspirin intolerant asthmatic patients: a pilot study. *Thorax* **43**:93–97.

Rosenstein, E.D., Kushner, L.J., Kramer, N., and Kazandjian, G. 2003. Pilot study of dietary fatty acid supplementation in the treatment of adult periodontitis. *Prostaglandins Leukot. Essent. Fatty Acids* **68**:213–218.

Simopoulos, A.P. 2002. Omega-3 fatty acids in inflammation and autoimmune diseases. *J. Am. Coll. Nutr.* **21**:495–505.

Spector, S.L., Surette, M.E. 2003. Diet and asthma: has the role of dietary lipids been overlooked in the management of asthma? *Ann. Allergy Asthma Immunol.* **90(4)**:371–377.

Surette, M.E., Koumenis, I.L., Edens, M.B., Tramposch, K.M., and Chilton, F.H. 2003. Inhibition of leukotriene synthesis, pharmacokinetics, and tolerability of a novel dietary fatty acid formulation in healthy adult subjects. *Clin. Ther.* **25**:948–971.

Surette, M.E., Edens, M., Chilton, F.H., and Tramposch, K.M. 2004. Dietary echium oil increases plasma and neutrophil long-chain (n-3) fatty acids and lowers serum triacylglycerols in hypertriglyceridemic humans. *J. Nutr.* **134**:1406–1411.

Thien, F.C.K., Atkinson, B.A., Khan, A., Mencia-Huerta, J.-M., and Lee, T.H. 1992. Effect of dietary fish oil supplementation on the antigen-induced late-phase response in the skin. *J. Allergy Clin. Immunol.* **89**:829–835.

Thien, F.C.K., Menciahuerta, J.M., and Lee, T.K. 1993. Dietary fish oil: effects on seasonal hay fever and asthma in pollen-sensitive subjects. *Am. Rev. Respir. Dis.* **147**:1138–1143.

Tollesson, A., and Frithz, A. 1993. Borage oil, an effective new treatment for infantile seborrhoeic dermatitis. *Br. J. Dermatol.* **129**:95.

Ursin, V.M. 2003. Modification of plant lipids for human health: development of functional land-based omega-3 fatty acids. *J. Nutr.* **133**:4271–4274.

van Gool, C.J., Thijs, C., Henquet, C.J., van Houwelingen, A.C., Dagnelie, P.C., Schrander, J., Menheere, P.P., and van den Brandt, P.A. 2003. Gamma-linolenic acid supplementation for prophylaxis of atopic dermatitis—a randomized controlled trial in infants at high familial risk. *Am. J. Clin. Nutr.* **77**:943–951.

Wensing, A.G., Mensink, R.P., and Hornstra, G. 1999. Effects of dietary n-3 polyunsaturated fatty acids from plant and marine origin on platelet aggregation in healthy elderly subjects. *Br. J. Nutr.* **82**:183–191.

Chapter 10: What's Your I.Q.?

Berry, K.A., Borgeat, P., Gosselin, J., Flamand, L., and Murphy, R.C. 2003. Urinary metabolites of leukotriene B_4 in the human subject. *J. Biol. Chem.* **278**:24449–24460.

Christie, P.E., Tagari, P., Ford-Hutchinson, A.W., Charlesson, S., Chee, P., Arm, J.P., and Lee, T.H. 1991. Urinary leukotriene E_4 concentrations increase after aspirin challenge in aspirin-sensitive asthmatic subjects. *Am. Rev. Respir. Dis.* **143**:1025–1029.

Drazen, J.M., O'Brien, J., Sparrow, D., Weiss, S.T., Martins, M.A., Israel, E., and Fanta, C.H. 1992. Recovery of leukotriene E_4 from the urine of patients with airway obstruction. *Am. Rev. Respir. Dis.* **146**:104–108.

Smith, C.M., Christie, P.E., Hawksworth, R.J., Thien, F., and Lee, T.H. 1991. Urinary leukotriene E_4 levels following allergen and exercise challenge in bronchial asthma. *Am. Rev. Respir. Dis.* **144**:1411–1413.

Smith, C.M., Hawksworth, R.J., Thien, F.C.K., Christie, P.E., and Lee, T.H. 1992. Urinary leukotriene E_4 in bronchial asthma. *Eur. Respir. J.* **5**:693–699.

Taylor, G.W., Taylor, I., Black, P., Maltby, N.H., Turner, N., Fuller, R.W., and

Dollery, C.T. 1989. Urinary leukotriene E_4 after antigen challenge and in acute asthma and allergic rhinitis. *Lancet* **1**:584–588.

Westcott, J.Y., Smith, H.R., Wenzel, S.E., Larsen, G.L., Thomas, R.B., Felsien, D., and Voelkel, N.F. 1991. Urinary leukotriene E_4 in patients with asthma: effect of airways reactivity and sodium cromoglycate. *Am. Rev. Respir. Dis.* **143**:1322–1328.

Yeh, E.T. 2004. C-reactive protein is an essential aspect of cardiovascular risk factor stratification. *Can. J. Cardiol.* **20**:93B–96B.

Yeh, E.T. 2004. CRP as a mediator of disease. *Circulation* **109**:II11–II14.

Index

About the Authors

FLOYD H. "SKI" CHILTON, PH.D., is widely recognized in academia and industry for his work on the role of fatty acids in human disease. Dr. Chilton also has extensive experience in leading organizations in both academia and industry. Dr. Chilton is currently a full professor in the Department of Physiology and Pharmacology at Wake Forest University School of Medicine. Prior to joining Wake Forest, Dr. Chilton founded a biotechnology company, Pilot Therapeutics, and served as its President, CEO, and Chief Technology Officer from late 2000 to 2003. At Pilot Therapeutics, Dr. Chilton is currently overseeing development of a medical food called Airozin, which blocks inflammatory messengers that cause asthma and arthritis. In 2003, Dr. Chilton was named an Ernst and Young Entrepreneur of the Year Finalist for the Carolinas (one of three finalists selected from more than four hundred CEOs in North and South Carolina in the Biotechnology/Life Sciences category).

Prior to founding Pilot Therapeutics, Dr. Chilton founded the Program in Molecular Medicine at Wake Forest University School of Medicine and helped build it into one of the most successful programs of its kind in the United States. During his time at Wake Forest, Dr. Chilton has served as Director of Molecular Medicine, Professor of Physiology and Pharmacology, Professor of Internal Medicine, and Professor of Biochemistry; and he has also served as Associate Director of the Asthma and Airways Diseases Center and Associate Director of Programs in Clinical Research. Prior to Wake Forest, Dr. Chilton served on the faculty at Johns Hopkins School of Medicine.

Dr. Chilton holds thirty-two issued and seventeen pending patents. He has authored or coauthored more than 110 scientific articles and book chapters. Dr. Chilton has served as chairman of, and organizer of, several international meetings on dietary regulation of human disease and lipid metabolism. Dr. Chilton obtained his Ph.D. in biochemistry from Wake Forest University in 1984. He served as a postdoctoral fellow in pharmacology at the University of Colorado until 1986. He has received numerous awards during his career, including the Cowgill Scholar Award and the Sigma Xi Research Award at Wake Forest, the

1999 Distinguished Academic and Achievement Award from Western Carolina University, and the Distinguished Service and Teaching Award from the Italian Congress on Allergy and Immunology.

CHARLES E. "CASH" McCALL, M.D, is Professor of Internal Medicine, Microbiology, and Immunology; Director of the General Clinical Research Center; and Deputy Associated Dean for Research at Wake Forest University Health Sciences. Dr. McCall received his M.D. degree as the top academic graduate of 1961 from what is now known as the Wake Forest University School of Medicine (WFUSM). After five years of postgraduate training at Harvard Medical School and two years at the Centers for Disease Control (CDC), he returned as a faculty member at WFUSM in 1968. In 1972, during the early stages of Dr. McCall's career at WFUBMC, he held an NIH Research Career Development Award and a Postgraduate Medical Fellowship assigned to research at the Royal Postgraduate School of Medicine in London. He was Director of the Division of Infectious Diseases, 1973–1998, Acting Chairman of Microbiology and Immunology, 1981–1983, and he served as Vice Chair of the Department of Internal Medicine for Research and Academic Affairs for eleven years. He has been Director of the NIH-funded General Clinical Research Center (GCRC) since its inception in 1993.

Dr. McCall was the first member of the faculty of WFUSM to be elected to the American Society of Clinical Investigation and the Association of American Physicians.

Dr. McCall has dedicated most of his career to translational clinical research in inflammation, and he is an author of over 160 original research publications. He has been consistently funded for inflammation research since 1970. His successful career in translational patient-oriented research in inflammation led to his being awarded the first Established Investigator Award in Clinical Research at Wake Forest University Medical School in 1997. Dr. McCall is also the recipient of the Distinguished Faculty Alumnus Award and the Distinguished Service Award of Wake Forest University School of Medicine.

LAURA TUCKER has written several popular health and medical books. She lives with her husband and daughter in Brooklyn, New York.